KV-281-810

Contents

Preface

When David Crystal suggested that I undertake to produce a book which could explain the vocabulary of alternative and complementary medicine I was pleased to accept the challenge, thinking:

(1) that the topic was far less daunting than attempting to compile a medical dictionary;

(2) whereas there are several excellent medical dictionaries available, there is no equivalent 'alternative' compilation of which I am aware;

(3) that in the process I would add to my knowledge of this rapidly expanding field in which I have developed an absorbing and increasing interest.

That thought (3) has proved to be true is beyond question, and thought (2) I believe still to be the case, although the bibliography is expanding rapidly. Thought (1) I now realize was a definite misconception.

The choice which faces the seeker after alternative or complementary therapy in the UK in 1993 is now quite bewildering. Exotic therapies, some with their origins disappearing into antiquity, have been imported from all around the world, and at the same time new systems of treatment are ever in the process of development. Sometimes these new treatments have been developed by combining aspects of already well-established systems, and sometimes they are based on entirely new concepts of health and pathology which have yet to stand the tests of time and critical appraisal.

As new concepts and therapies proliferate, their growth is paralleled by an uncontrolled expansion of the terminology. Neologisms abound, sometimes because their originators are unaware of identical concepts already described in other sister disciplines with which they, themselves, are unfamiliar. If a subject is constrained by the discipline of objective and precise methods of observation (eg physics) then usually one word suffices to describe one concept. In a chaotic system where each event is described from multiple parochial viewpoints and where there has been no organized attempt to standardize

Making Sense of
English in

Alternative
Medicine

Peter Gravett

Chambers

Published 1993 by Chambers Harrap Publishers Ltd
43–45 Annandale Street, Edinburgh EH7 4AZ

A catalogue record for this book is available from the
British Library

ISBN 0 550 18047 8

Other titles in the series:

Making Sense of English Usage
Making Sense of Foreign Words in English
Making Sense of English in Money Matters
Making Sense of English in the Law
Making Sense of English in Religion
Making Sense of English in Sex
Making Sense of English in Computers
Making Sense of English in Psychology

Typeset by Pillans & Wilson Ltd, Edinburgh
Printed in England by Clays Ltd, St Ives plc

vocabulary, an independent observer has no way of choosing between several apparently equally applicable words. Faced with this situation, I have taken the example of David Crystal in his original book of this series, *Making Sense of English Usage*, and produced an anthology — a limited and personal selection of words and terms which I have encountered, found to be of interest, and attempted to define to my own satisfaction. Many of the entries include information beyond that required of a dictionary definition, which may reflect my own particular enthusiasms. I have limited the inclusion of synonyms to avoid an enormous amount of cross-referencing and a substantial increase in the size of this volume.

The sources of information from which this anthology was compiled are many and varied. Some well-established therapies have recognized text books which are used as the basis for training courses that lead to formal qualifications, but many other emerging disciplines have, as yet, only magazine articles and information leaflets from which to glean details. I have acquired much information, and derived considerable enjoyment, from attending meetings and exhibitions such as the Alternative Health Exhibition at Olympia, and the Mind, Body, Spirit Festival which happens over the Spring Bank Holiday each year. Such events are an unfailing source of leaflets, as well as giving an opportunity for direct discussion with practitioners and, even better, the opportunity to sample the therapies personally. The excellent *Journal of Alternative and Complementary Medicine* has introduced me to many words that I would not otherwise have encountered, and to the writings of many of today's leading practitioners on both sides of the Atlantic divide. I have also been fortunate in being allowed to use the facilities of two of London's leading complementary centres, the Hale Clinic and the Marylebone Health Centre in Regent's Park. So many individuals have helped with compiling and producing this volume that it would be impractical to list them individually, but I am nevertheless sincerely grateful for the generous assistance, from every direction, that I have been offered and glad to accept.

This volume makes no attempt to provide a comprehensive catalogue of available therapies, and as a dictionary it is even less complete. Some of the entries do not constitute formal definitions, but rather offer information and clarification of the use and meaning of each word or term. The inclusion of a particular therapy should in no way be taken as an endorsement of its validity. I have deliberately surveyed as wide a range of topics as possible, some of which could reasonably be thought of as 'orthodox', many as unorthodox, and some that I believe a well-informed and unbiased observer would reasonably classify as unmitigated nonsense. My objective has not been to enable my reader to make a selection from the myriad of therapies available, but rather to attempt to explain some of the vocabulary likely to be encountered in the search.

As an orthodox medical practitioner with a long-established interest in martial arts, traditional Chinese medicine, and acupuncture, I feel that I should add a final word on the distinction between *alternative* and *complementary* medicine. *Complementary medicine* is a term which embraces a huge variety of treatment systems which aim to work alongside orthodox medicine so that the two systems together cooperate for the benefit of the patient. *Alternative medicine* implies that there is direct competition with the orthodox approach without entertaining the possibility of interaction between them. Whereas I do not doubt that, in some circumstances, alternative treatments can claim as much or even more success than their orthodox equivalent, I believe that the danger of inappropriate measures being applied, or of essential orthodox treatment being delayed or even withheld in cases of serious illness, should not be underestimated. The complementary approach is not only safer for all concerned, but I believe will prove in the long run to be to the benefit of both patients and practitioners.

As alternative and complementary medicine become more popular, there will be an ever-increasing number of practitioners, practising an ever-increasing number of therapies. Many of the major therapies have, by now, formed professional organizations with well defined philosophies, objectives, and standards required of their members. These associations produce lists of accredited practitioners who are required to show a certain minimum level of competence before they can be accepted for registration, and some of the qualifications listed in the Appendix are obtained only after an extended course of study with searching examinations that must be passed before the qualification is awarded. Such qualifications have national recognition and are widely respected. Unfortunately some of the other 'qualifications' listed are no more than in-house certificates of attendance at courses, awarded by self-appointed authorities, in subjects which have no objective basis for independent assessment and which may be completely worthless in terms of treatment and healing.

In swimming through this sea of alternative and complementary practitioners the reader should not necessarily be impressed by lists of letters following a therapist's name. The letters have only as much credibility as the organizations which grant them and, unless backed by a reputable organization, cannot be taken as any sort of guarantee either of the validity of the treatment offered or of the competence of the individual practitioner. In the field of natural healing it may well be that some of the most effective practitioners claim no formal qualifications, and indeed the effectiveness of an individual practitioner may even prove to be inversely proportional to the number of letters listed after his or her name.

Peter Gravett

Pronunciation Guide

Vowels

iː	need	/niːd/
ɪ	pit	/pɪt/
i	very	/ˈvɛri/
ɛ	pet	/pɛt/
æ	pat	/pæt/
ʌ	other	/ˈʌðəʳ/
ʊ	book	/bʊk/
uː	too	/tuː/
u	influence	/ˈɪnfluəns/
ɒ	cough	/kɒf/
ɔː	ought	/ɔːt/
ɜː	work	/wɜːk/
ə	another	/əˈnʌðəʳ/
ɑː	part	/pɑːt/

Glides

eɪ	plate	/pleɪt/
aɪ	sigh	/saɪ/
ɔɪ	ploy	/plɔɪ/
oʊ	go	/goʊ/
aʊ	now	/naʊ/
ɪə	hear	/hɪəʳ/
ɛə	fair	/fɛəʳ/
ʊə	poor	/pʊəʳ/

Consonants

p	pit	/pɪt/
b	bit	/bɪt/
t	ten	/tɛn/
d	den	/dɛn/
k	cap	/kæp/
g	gap	/gæp/
ʃ	shin	/ʃɪn/
ʒ	pleasure	/ˈplɛʒəʳ/
ʧ	chin	/ʧɪn/
ʤ	budge	/bʌʤ/
h	hit	/hɪt/
f	fit	/fɪt/
v	very	/ˈvɛri/
θ	thin	/θɪn/
ð	then	/ðɛn/
s	sin	/sɪn/
z	zones	/zoʊnz/
m	meat	/miːt/
n	knit	/nɪt/
ŋ	sing	/sɪŋ/
l	line	/laɪn/
r	rid	/rɪd/
j	yet	/jɛt/
w	quick	/kwɪk/

Foreign sound

ã	French *temps*	/tã/

Other symbols

ʳ indicates an 'r' pronounced only before a following vowel
ˈ precedes the syllable with primary stress

Note

Words or phrases within an entry that are printed in **bold type** refer the reader to another entry where there is further relevant information. *Italic type* is used within entries to indicate significant related words that do not themselves have an entry (although they may have a cross-reference). Sources of words are also shown in italic type.

A

absent healing

A method of treatment which does not require the patient's presence (or participation) for its application. For example, practitioners of **spiritual healing** may use prayer and meditation to activate a patient's own healing powers, or a **radionics** instrument may be used to transmit healing energies to a patient. This is particularly useful for the very young, very old, and those too ill to travel for their treatment.

See also **healing**

acidophilus /æsɪˈdɒfɪləs/

Lactobacillus acidophilus is a 'probiotic' or friendly bacterium used to colonize the gut, especially when it has been upset by a poor diet, antibiotic therapy, or intercurrent illness. It may be taken in the form of a dietary supplement to reduce the hazard from pathogenic bacteria, yeasts, and fungi such as **candida**.

See also **probiotics; yoghurt**

acquired immunodeficiency syndrome
See **AIDS**

acupressure

The application of pressure to **acupuncture** points, using thumb and fingertip pressure, to stimulate the body's own healing powers. It may also include massaging along the direction of the acupuncture **meridians** with short rapid movements to stimulate and balance the flow of **qi**.

See also **shiatsu, shen tao** and **jin shin do**, which have the same origins.

acupuncture

[Latin *acus* 'needle' + *punctura* 'a piercing'] An ancient Chinese healing art in which fine needles are inserted into precise points in the body. These points are located on **meridians** through which **qi** energy flows and through which they are linked to internal organs. Diagnosis is based on **traditional Chinese medicine** in which illness is seen as an imbalance of energy or blockage in energy flow. The object of acupuncture is to correct these imbalances and restore the flow of **qi** energy through the **meridians**. This may involve using electricity, laser, magnetism, or heat as well as needle puncture techniques.

adaptogen

A substance (eg a herb such as **eleutherococcus senticosus**) which helps to maintain the systems by which the body adapts to changes in its internal environment and maintains its physiological balance even in the presence of adverse factors such as infection, radiation, or toxins.

addiction

Dependence upon a substance without which the addict's body cannot function normally. Addictive substances alter the body chemistry and lead to a continual craving which usually requires increasing amounts of the substance to maintain the same level of effect (this is known as **tolerance**). As the body becomes dependent on the presence of an addictive substance, the addict will suffer **withdrawal** symptoms unless adequate supplies of the substance are maintained. Smoking, alcohol, and tranquillizers are addictive, as are the so-called 'hard' drugs.

aerobics

An exercise, or series of exercises, made popular in the 1980s as a means of attaining and maintaining physical fitness. The exercises are often performed to music, and are sufficiently vigorous to increase the body's need for oxygen and hence the air intake and breathing rate. They are intended to produce cardio-vascular stress, and the effect is assessed by taking the

pulse rate before and after each exercise programme, with targets being set according to the age of the participant and the type of exertion being practised.
See also **anaerobic**

agrimony

A perennial plant from which a **Bach flower remedy** can be extracted which is said to help those people who hide their worries behind a cheerful face. The remedy helps them to relax, share their problems, and put their difficulties into perspective.

AIDS

Acquired immunodeficiency syndrome, a failure of the immune system which is the late end result of infection by the Human Immunodeficiency Virus (**HIV**). This destroys some of the body's lymphocytes, and consequently its ability to resist infection even by organisms which do not usually cause disease. Cancers such as lymphomas and Kaposi's Sarcoma, which may themselves have a viral origin, may also occur.
See also **immune system**

aikido

A Japanese martial art developed by Mori Ueshiba (1883–1969) which emphasizes the 'way of spiritual harmony' and the use of body movements to neutralize and redirect the force of an attacker. The art is non-competitive and non-aggressive, but is very effective both as a form of exercise and as a system of self-defence.

air imbalance

A lack of balance between negative and positive charged particles in the air caused by **electro-pollution**, which may have adverse effects on health leading to headaches and impaired concentration. Fresh air usually contains five positive particles to every four negative particles, and imbalance may be corrected by using an **ionizer**.

ajna /ˈɑːdʒnə/

The sixth **chakra** situated in the centre of the forehead, corresponding to the 'third eye' or pineal gland which is situated deep in the brain, above the third ventricle, and which synthesizes the hormone melatonin. This chakra is said to be the centre of psychic activity, the seat of 'second sight', and to influence sleep, clarity of thought, and general energy levels. It is considered to be the 'command' chakra.

Alexander technique

A technique of posture training developed by the Australian actor F Matthias Alexander (1869–1955) which was designed to encourage people to rediscover their natural posture and movement and to discard harmful and unnatural habitual postures that they have acquired. This is said to lead to a general improvement of neuromuscular coordination with reduction in physical and mental tension. It is increasingly popular as a therapy for headaches, backaches, anxiety, and depression, and particularly benefits stage performers such as actors, musicians, and dancers.

alfalfa

A perennial plant with purple flowers (*Medicago sativa*), first cultivated in ancient Persia as a forage crop, and called 'the father of foods' by the Arabs; also known as *lucerne*. Its roots extend as much as 30ft into the earth extracting nutrients that other plants cannot reach, and it is widely used as a dietary supplement, containing many enzymes including lipase, amylase, and proteinases.

allergy

An abnormal reaction of the body's immune system to a foreign substance (the *allergen*) which results in the release of inflammation-producing substances including histamine, hydroxytryptamine, and bradykinin. Virtually any substance can act as an allergen to which the body's immune system can become sensitized. Subsequent exposure to minute amounts of this substance may provoke reactions such as skin rashes following direct contact (eg certain plants), asthma or allergic

rhinitis (eg pollen and dust mites), nausea, vomiting, or diarrhoea (eg dairy products, shell fish).
See also **allergy therapy, cytotoxic testing, elimination diet, food allergy**

allergy therapy
A therapy which identifies the substances producing an illness by provoking an allergic reaction and then providing specific treatment to neutralize the allergic response. Many common foods act as allergens and produce a wide range of symptoms, including gastro-intestinal problems, headache, depression, and arthritis. The most frequently implicated allergens are white flour, dairy products, and food additives. Diagnosis is made by identifying the allergens responsible for the symptoms by using blood testing, scratch testing, or an exclusion diet. Treatment involves avoiding the precipitating allergen, or *desensitization* by injection of diluted allergen to build **tolerance**.
See also **allergy**

allopathy
[Greek *allos* 'different' + *pathos* 'suffering'] A descriptive term for conventional or orthodox medicine, coined by Samuel Hahnemann (the German physician who developed **homeopathy**). Allopathic medicine employs treatment to suppress the symptoms of an illness using the principle of opposites, eg analgesics for pain, sedatives for sleeplessness, purgatives for constipation. This is in contrast to homeopathy, which sees the symptoms as expressions of the body's reaction to disease, which are to be encouraged rather than suppressed.

alternative medicine
A general term encompassing those therapies which can be used as an alternative to (ie instead of) conventional or orthodox Western medicine. Many of these are empirical, but are based upon long-established systems of diagnosis and treatment, such as **traditional Chinese medicine**, which can claim results at least as effective as the scientific medical approach, especially for the treatment of chronic pain, degenerative disease, and stress-related illnesses. With

increasing public interest in these methods, some alternative treatments are being adopted by conventional medical practitioners, and trials are now being conducted to allow proper scientific appraisal of their effectiveness.

See also **complementary medicine**

amalgam toxicity

A type of poisoning which results from mercury amalgam dental fillings which emit toxic vapour from their surface. This is up to 50 times more marked with the recent 'high copper' type fillings than from conventional amalgams. Mercury vapour emission produces a form of heavy metal poisoning which causes non-specific symptoms, so that 77% of patients complain of chronic fatigue and 60% of un-explained irritability and anger. 90% of these patients show improvement in symptoms after their amalgam is removed.

amber

A solidified resin from pine trees which often contains visible parts of insects. It may be worn as jewellery or decoration, and is said to bring life-giving energy from the sun, to absorb negativity, and to balance **yin** and **yang**.

See also **crystal therapy**

amethyst

An indigo-violet stone, associated with the third eye **chakra**, which has a reputation as a healing gem and spiritual stone, also associated with intuition and spiritual awakening. It is said to calm passion, violence, and anger, and to promote chastity and sleep.

See also **crystal therapy**

AMI

An **A**pparatus developed in 1975 for measuring the func-tioning of the **M**eridians and their corresponding **I**nternal organs, invented by Dr Hiroshi Motoyama (1925–   ), a Japanese parapsychologist, scientist and Shinto priest. The apparatus is claimed to demonstrate the acupuncture meridians on screen, and to measure the flow of energy within each meridian, relating this to the functioning of the internal organs.

anaerobic

[Literally 'without air or oxygen'] A term applied to microbes which can thrive only in the absence of oxygen. It also refers to the converse of **aerobic** exercise, where sustained intensive exercise (eg sprinting) exceeds the body's capacity to deliver oxygen, so that the muscles use energy derived from anaerobic metabolism resulting in an oxygen deficit which has to be replenished later.

See also **aerobics**

anahata /ænəˈhætə/

The fourth **chakra**, or heart chakra, which is situated behind the heart and linked with the cardiac plexus. It corresponds with the cardio-vascular system as well as having some effect on the small intestine, and is also concerned with skin touch and feelings which are manifested in art, poetry, and music.

analytical trilogy

A concept developed to integrate the three essential aspects of a human being, ie feelings, thought, and action, which correspond to theology, philosophy, and science.

See also **integral psychoanalysis**

animal game

A bioenergetic exercise in which group members choose an animal with which they can identify, imitating its posture and behaviour. Subsequent discussion by the group, under the guidance of a therapist, may allow a new or deeper understanding of personal relationships and behaviour.

See also **bioenergetics**

an mo /ˈɑːn ˈmoʊ/

A Chinese system of remedial massage dating from the Han period in which pressing and rubbing specific body areas tonifies the corresponding internal organs.

See also **tui na**

anthroposophical medicine

[Greek *anthropos* 'man'+*sophia* 'wisdom'] A medical philosophy developed by Rudolph Steiner (1861–1925), recognizing that people, life, and illness cannot be completely understood just by the physical senses alone. He saw people as consisting of four inter-related but independent 'bodies':

1 physical body — the basic structure;
2 etheric body — living and full of creative force;
3 astral body — consisting of driving force and emotions;
4 consciousness of self as a being — the spiritual dimension.

Illness was seen as a malfunction of all four bodies, but also as an opportunity to overcome imbalances and correct harmful ways of living. Since emotions are so important in maintaining health, Steiner taught that physical treatments must be backed up by treatment of the mind to maintain the balance between mind and body. He sympathized with homeopathic principles, and emphasized the value of plants as medicines, since they concentrate minerals and cosmic forces.

antioxidants

Chemicals which have a protective effect by neutralizing **free radicals** which have been implicated in tissue damage and in causing cancer. Vitamins A, C, and E and carotene have been shown to be beneficial in treating rheumatoid arthritis, hypertension, and Parkinson's disease, and also in protecting against carcinoma of the mouth, oesophagus, stomach, and rectum. Enzyme preparations from wheat sprouts such as SOD/CAT or AOX/PLX can be taken in tablet form as a dietary supplement, and have been used to suppress musculo-skeletal and synovial inflammation in treating various forms of arthritis.

aphrodisiac

A substance said to stimulate or enhance sexual desire. Examples include foods such as oysters and nasturtium leaves, essential oils such as jasmine, patchouli oil, and ylang ylang, herbs such as ginseng, and concoctions such as powdered rhinoceros horn and *Spanish Fly*, which consists of crushed dried beetles.

apitherapy

The use of honey bee products to treat disease and promote health, for example **royal jelly** and **propolis**. These are nutritious natural health foods, rich in vitamins and trace elements, which may be useful as a dietary supplement, and which some people believe have other, less tangible, beneficial effects.

aquamarine

A clear blue stone, also known as the 'water' stone, which is said to prevent negative thinking, to eliminate excess fluid from the body, and to clear the glands and the nervous system.
See also **crystal therapy**

aromatherapy

The use of highly concentrated essential oils extracted from plants as a form of therapy. Therapists use various systems such as conventional medicine, **traditional Chinese medicine** or **radiesthesia** to establish a diagnosis and select essential oils. Oils may be used topically (eg eucalyptus as an antiseptic, clove oil for toothache) or they may be applied by massage. Application to the skin is a very effective way of getting active agents into the blood stream. They are then distributed throughout the extra-cellular fluid, some being concentrated in specific organs. Oils may also be inhaled using a vaporizer or taken internally by mouth, or as a suppository or pessary.

Clinical aromatherapy may be viewed as a branch of **herbal medicine**, and some oils have good antiseptic, antibacterial, antifungal, and antiviral properties. *Cosmetic aromatherapy* is offered by many beauty salons, usually using pre-blended oils.

artemesia

Artemesia vulgaris, otherwise known as the common mugwort or Chinese wormwood. The dried leaves of this plant are used to produce **moxa**, which is used in **moxibustion** to apply external heat, particularly in the treatment of damp and cold conditions.

art therapy

A type of therapy which was introduced to England during the 1940s as a result of the work of the artist Adrian Hill and the psychotherapist Irene Champernowne. It is a combination of the visual arts (such as painting and collage) with psychotherapy, and is used, particularly in psychiatric hospitals, to help patients who find it difficult to express themselves. Art therapy allows self-expression through drawing and painting, and this releases emotional tension. An art therapist may be able to interpret the meaning of a painting to give insight about patients, their life, and even the contents of their subconscious mind.

asoene /æsoʊˈiːn/

A constituent of **garlic** which can be extracted in a pure form, and which has been shown to kill certain cancer (lymphoma) cells.

aspen

A species of poplar from the leaves of which a **Bach flower remedy** can be extracted. This is said to help those people who are excessively apprehensive and who suffer attacks of panic and fear for no apparent reason.

assertion training

A form of **behaviour therapy** designed to enable patients to develop social skills in which they feel deficient, particularly to practise standing up for their own rights in specific situations that they find difficult. It includes three main elements:

1 skills training — verbal and non-verbal behaviour practised by role play which emphasizes assertive behaviour;
2 methods for reducing anxiety, such as relaxation exercises;
3 examining and discussing values and beliefs about the rights of the individual in society.

aura

The energy field radiating from a living organism (both plants and animals), which some people can sense directly but which may also be viewed using a **Kilner screen** or demonstrated by **Kirlian photography**. The shape, colour and strength of an aura varies with the individual, and is affected by sickness, health, and activity. An aura interacts with other auras in the vicinity, and a therapist may be able to detect ill health in specific organs from its appearance.

auricular cardiac reflex

A clinical test which relies on the shape of the arterial pulse wave, usually taken at the radial pulse, to assess the response to contact with a food, chemical or other allergen to which the body may be sensitive.
See also **allergy**

auricular therapy *or* auriculotherapy

A form of **acupuncture** using points in the ear. It is particularly used to treat addictions, including those to alcohol, drugs, food, and tobacco, and for pain relief during childbirth and dentistry. The ear has more than 200 acupuncture points described, which are physically related to particular areas of the body. The position of these points roughly corresponds to the image of an inverted foetus over the surface of the ear, and they were described in classical Chinese texts. A detailed ear map was developed by Dr Paul Nogier in France in 1951. Giving treatment to these points by needling, electronic stimulation, or laser may cure disease in related organs.

autogenic training

[Greek *auto* 'self' + *genic* 'producing'] A form of training which involves self-hypnosis by concentrating on the breathing or on tensions within the body. This induces a hypnotic state somewhere between full consciousness and sleep, which allows access to the unconscious mind. Visual exercises, such as recalling incidents from the past, are performed, and pleasant incidents can be anchored in the memory. A series of six mental exercises are described which are aimed at relieving stress and helping the body to cure itself by changing unwanted behaviour patterns. This technique is useful for people who have difficulty with relaxing, and who suffer tension-induced problems such as headaches and colitis.

autosuggestion

A form of meditation, also known as **Couéism**, which is designed to empty the mind of conscious thought by the repetition of a word or phrase (**mantra**). With the mind in a relaxed state, behaviour patterns may be influenced through the unconscious, and the healing powers of the body and mind released.

aversion therapy

A form of **behaviour therapy** in which an unwanted response is associated with an unpleasant stimulus. This has been called 'learning by punishment' (eg by receiving electric shocks), and requires both the patient's cooperation and a genuine desire to change their behaviour. Some drug treatments for alcoholism result in violent sickness on taking alcohol.

awareness through movement

A technique to make people aware of their habitual movement patterns and the possibilities for changing them. The term is applied to group lessons rather than individual therapy.
See also **Feldenkrais method**

ayurveda

[Hindu *ayur* 'life' + *veda* 'knowledge, science'] A sacred system of medicine from ancient India which still plays an important part in the Far East. Good health is thought of as the result of three forces being in harmony:

1 *vata* (air), which governs movement (equivalent to psycho-motor activity);
2 *pitta* (fire), which governs digestion and warmth (equivalent to metabolic activity);
3 *kapha* (water), which governs cohesion and lubrication (equivalent to the growth aspects of life).

Wrong food, physical activity, sex, climate, emotional state, and environment can all influence the onset of disease, and each person is considered unique and subject to unique imbalances. A history is taken which includes astrological assessment, and emphasis is placed both on a doctrine of prevention (ie treating a disease before it actually appears) and on the patient's own obligation to be obedient to any instruction and to play their own part in curing their illness. The treatment may include fasting, bathing, diets, and enemas to clean the body prior to giving more specific therapy. There is a large herbal pharmocopeia used to balance body systems, and massage, prayers, and yogic breathing may also be employed.

B

Bach flower remedies /bɑːk/

One in a system of floral remedies, claimed to affect the emotional state, developed by Edward Bach (1880–1936). They are prepared from 38 species of flower indigenous to the United Kingdom. The original belief was that warm dew would absorb the properties of a plant from whose surface it was collected, and could then be taken by mouth as a treatment for various disorders. The remedies are now produced as a simple aqueous extract, but with small quantities of brandy added as a preservative. They may be used for self-treatment, particularly for anxiety and negative emotional states, and prescription is according to one's temperament and personality. A combination of five of the 38 remedies is recommended as a cure-all for any emergency situation, available under the name of **rescue remedy**.

Bates' method

A series of exercises developed by Dr William H Bates (1860–1931) to improve and maintain healthy eyesight without the use of spectacles; also called *eye therapy*. He published a book in 1919 entitled *Better Eyesight Without Glasses*, explaining poor sight as a disturbance of normal mind-body coordination which may result from mental, emotional, or other disturbances. Exercises in relaxation, memory, imagination, and perception improve the feedback between the eyes and the brain.

bathing

See **hydrotherapy** and **thalassotherapy**

becquerel

A unit of radioactivity which includes the activity of **radon** gas. The name derives from Antoine Henri Becquerel (1852–1908), a French physicist who won the Nobel Prize for Physics in 1903 (with the Curies).

beech

A deciduous tree, found in Great Britain, with tiny flowers which can be used to prepare a **Bach flower remedy** to help people who are critical and intolerant of others to be more understanding. People with this type of personality consider themselves to be perfectionists, and are annoyed by other people's idiosyncracies.

behaviour therapy *or* behavioural therapy

A type of psychotherapy developed by Joseph Wolpe (1915–) which is based on the premise that behaviour is something that is learned as a response to the environment. People modify their behaviour to suit their circumstances, and undesirable behaviour can be unlearned and replaced by something better. This process usually involves the clinical use of **biofeedback**, possibly using a system of punishment or reward under the guidance of a clinical psychologist or psychotherapist. It has been used successfully to treat stress-related illness by introducing various forms of relaxation, but it is essential that patients are well-motivated and accept responsibility for the management of their own illness, as long-term success often requires a complete modification of lifestyle.

See also **flooding**

Benveniste theory /bãvəni:st/

A theory that molecules have 'memories', published by French scientist Jacques Benveniste in 1988. He performed a series of experiments at INSERM (the French Medical Research Council in Paris) in which he claimed to prove that an antibody solution, repeatedly diluted until no more molecules of antibody could be present, could still provoke a detectable response from white blood cells. This demonstration, if confirmed by other workers, would clearly support one of the fundamental tenets of **homeopathy**.

Beres drops /'bɛrɛs/
A dietary supplement, developed by Hungarian biochemist Dr Josef Beres, which consists of a complex cocktail of trace elements including boron, cobalt, manganese, copper, iron, potassium, magnesium, nickel, vanadium, zinc, and molybdenum. It is supplied as a liquid to be taken by mouth to correct any deficiencies and allow optimal body function.

betony
A perennial plant related to the woundwort (*Stochys betonica*) with bright red flowers which contain the active principles (alkaloids) stacydrine, betonicine, and trigonelline. Although listed in the pharmacopoeia as a sedative, this herb is also useful as a tonic for those who are feeling run down or debilitated after illness.

biochemics
A system of treatment devised by a German homeopath, Dr Wilhelm Heinrich Schuessler (1821–1898) based on his belief that every form of illness is associated with an imbalance of the inorganic salts in the body. He developed a list of 12 essential 'tissue salts', and taught that the lack of a particular salt would cause specific symptoms. Subsequent research has expanded his original list to 30 essential trace elements, and commonly used combinations of these are freely available in pharmacies and health food shops for self-medication.

bioelectrography
A technique which uses a high-voltage electrical discharge system to investigate and record the luminosity of living tissues. This can give information about the functional state of the tissue, and attempts are being made to develop the method so that it is suitable for use in mass screening programmes for the early detection of cancer.
See also **Kirlian photography; bioluminescence**

bioelectrotherapy

A form of physical therapy in which a pad or membrane is applied to the skin over a diseased or injured area. The pad emits low energy electric current which is intended to activate the body's natural healing processes and accelerate pain relief. The apparatus was developed in 1988.

bioenergetics

A system of body orientated psychotherapy developed by Dr Alexander Lowen in the 1960s from the theories of Wilhelm Reich, who taught that body, mind, and feelings are all interrelated. It should thus be possible to deduce psychological and emotional problems from the posture and movements of the body (**body language**), and working on areas of tension using massage and exercises allows contact with the underlying emotions, relief of muscle tension, and the resumption of free and natural function.

See also **grounding**

biofeedback

An individual's ability to learn to control autonomic responses (ie those not usually under conscious control) by the use of appropriate monitoring devices. These include: sphygmomanometers and pulse meters, which allow training to reduce blood pressure; electro-encephalograms, which allow training to produce alpha brain waves (associated with well-being and relaxation); and various machines marketed as *relaxation meters*, which are said to be useful in treating stress-induced disorders and facilitating relaxation. *Feedback* is a method of controlling an inorganic system by re-inserting into it the results of its past performance. Biofeedback applies this same method to living systems.

See also **eclosion system**

bioholography

A technique based on the principle that each part of the body is thought to reflect the whole. For example **reflexology** depends upon the principle that the whole of the body is represented on the surface of the foot (mostly the soles of the feet) and that the internal organs can be stimulated by

bioluminescence

pressure on particular parts of the feet. **Auricular therapy** depends upon the image of the body being reflected on the surface of the ear. The analogy is with light holography, in which laser beams interact to produce a three-dimensional image, one characteristic of which is that the entire hologram can be reproduced from any small part of it.

bioluminescence

The energy created by cell metabolism, which causes molecular and electromagnetic vibrations covering the entire spectrum of electro-motive force (EMF) from extremely low frequency (ELF at 1 — 30 hertz) through to visible light. Most living organisms emit small amounts of light. Light may also be absorbed by living tissue from an external source and then re-emitted.

biomagnetics

A discipline which combines the principles of **acupuncture** and body magnetics. Illness is thought to result from an imbalance or block in the body's magnetic field, and may be treated by using small magnets placed on the body surface in positions corresponding to acupuncture points. This is said to be useful in the treatment of muscle and joint problems, anxiety and stress, fatigue and depression, and hormonal upsets including menopausal and premenstrual difficulties. See also **magnetic therapy**

bion /ˈbaɪɒn/

A unit of orgone energy.
See also **orgone therapy**

bionomy

A term referring to the two **biorhythms** which are represented by the male and female elements present in all cells and which influence features of behaviour. Austrian psychologist Herman Swoboda demonstrated c.1900 that the male nature has a 23-day cycle and the female nature a 28-day cycle. From these two rhythms a psychologist can predict periodic changes in behaviour and susceptibility to illness.

biorhythms

Physical, emotional, and intellectual cycles which affect human life and behaviour and which were charted by Wilhelm Fliess, Herman Swoboda and Alfred Teltscher during 1900–20; also referred to as *PSI theory*, from the three cycles involved. The Physical cycle is 23 days and governs vitality, strength, endurance, confidence, immunity, and sex drive. The Sensitivity or emotional cycle takes 28 days, and governs sensitivity, moods, nervous reactions, and creative ability. The Intellectual cycle spans 33 days, and governs memory, learning ability, and decision making. Since we are all subject to cyclical influences from the planets, the sun and solar system, the earth, and the moon, these factors interact to produce changes of mood, emotion, and susceptibility to illness.

The monthly periodicity of the menstrual cycle is an example of the body's cyclical variations, but orthodox medical science relates these changes to fluctuations in circulating hormone levels, and the various cycles that are defined do not coincide with the biorhythmic cycles described here.

These biorhythms may be calculated by extrapolating the various cycles from the date of birth, and this may allow understanding of behaviour patterns and warning of 'critical days' when one may expect exceptionally good or unavoidably poor performance.
See also **bionomy**

bi syndromes /biː/

In **traditional Chinese medicine** a blockage in the circulation of **qi** in the **meridians** which causes pain and stiffness in bones, joints, muscles, and tendons. This is traditionally seen as a response to invasion by wind, cold, or damp, resulting in five patterns of presentation: *wandering bi, painful bi, fixed bi, febrile bi,* and *bony bi*.

bloodstone

A form of iron ore (ferrous oxide) which is used for making jewellery because of its deep colour and lustre; also known as *haematite*. It is said to be good for blood-related disorders,

menstrual problems, and pregnancy. Legend says that bloodstone was formed when drops of Christ's blood fell to the earth from the cross and turned into stone.
See also **crystal therapy**

blue

A 'cool' colour which is associated with the sky, God, and heaven. It also relates to the throat **chakra**, and hence with speaking and communicating. Blue represents wisdom and truth, and has both antiseptic and soothing properties. Blue persons are idealistic, but have a tendency to be cool, passive, and indifferent.
See also **colour therapy**

body language

The use of body movement and posture to communicate without the use of spoken or written words. It may involve conscious actions, such as shaking hands or making gestures with socially recognizable meanings, or unconscious reactions such as blushing and blinking. The study of body language may give clues to a person's emotional state or to underlying tensions or psychological problems.
See also **bioenergetics; kinesics**

bodywork

A general term applied to those therapies which are designed to free and balance the body. There are four main types of technique:

1 *energetic* techniques relate to the vital energy systems such as **acupuncture** and **yoga**. This category might also include **faith healing**, which works by activating the body's own healing energies;
2 *mechanical* techniques include all forms of **massage** and manipulation, such as **rolfing** and the **Feldenkrais method**;
3 *psychological* techniques use the body to treat the mind and vice versa;
4 *integrative* techniques work on the links between physical, emotional, and mental balances, such as **tai chi chuan, yoga**

and **Heller work**. These all emphasize how to be whole, complete, and integrated in mind-body-spirit during the course of everyday life.

bone setter
A lay practitioner (ie a person with no formal medical education) using elementary techniques of manipulation to treat patients suffering skeletal injuries, particularly of the limbs, by repositioning bones that have been displaced by fracture or dislocation. The term dates from the 17th century.

boron
A rare non-metallic solid which does not occur naturally as a free element and which affects the bones. The average daily consumption in developing countries is 1–2 mg daily, but the use of chemical fertilizers, which prevent plants from extracting trace elements in the soil, is reducing the natural boron content of the diet. Supplements are now available which are said to diminish osteoporosis, neutralize the effects of excessive fluoridation, and improve symptoms in arthritis sufferers.

Bristol diet
A diet devised by Dr Alex Forbes, a founder member of the Bristol Cancer Help Centre, set up in 1979 to offer patients alternative therapies and treatments. The original principles were to begin with a low-fat, largely raw food, **vegan** diet, slowly introducing small amounts of vegetable oil, eggs, poultry, fish, etc as the patient's condition improved. More recently this has been modified to a basic whole-food diet with lots of fresh fruit and vegetables, whole grain, and pulses.

bromelain
See **pineapple**

bruxism
Tooth clenching and grinding. The problem affects one child in ten but usually disappears when the permanent teeth erupt. It is less common in adults, but is seen particularly in those who are compulsive overachievers, and also in people

with allergies (eg asthma, eczema, and hay fever sufferers). Sometimes it may be caused by dental problems such as missing teeth or badly fitting dentures, and it is also seen in patients with organic brain damage. The best forms of treatment include dental attention, stress reduction, **biofeedback, acupuncture,** and soft tissue techniques applied to **trigger points** around the head, neck, and jaw.

building biology

A science which examines the interaction between a building and its environment, emphasizing the effects of design features on the health of the occupants. The location and geometry of the building, its colour scheme, its lighting, and its furnishings will all affect its atmosphere. The use of non-toxic and ecologically friendly building materials will contribute further to the well-being of the occupants.

C

cabbage

A vegetable (*Brassica oleracea*) native to Europe and cultivated for its edible leaves, which are harvested before the
plant flowers. In alternative medicine it is widely used to treat
infection, particularly in Wales and East Anglia, where it may
be used, for example, as a poultice for applying to abscesses.
Cabbage juice is used in Ireland to treat sore throats,
hoarseness, and loss of voice. Cabbage water, with pepper
added, is used in Norfolk to treat cystitis. Crushed cabbage
leaves were used to treat foot and leg ulcers in the trenches of
the First World War.

caduceus /kæˈdjʊsiəs/

In classical mythology the wand carried by Mercury, the
messenger of the gods, which was said to have power over
health, happiness, sleep, and dreams. Because the staff
symbolized healing, it has been adopted by the medical
profession as their emblem. The caduceus is usually shown as
a central staff with two serpents entwined around it, crossing
at seven points down the length of the staff. These seven
intersections represent the seven **chakras**, with the third eye
being placed between the two serpent heads. The staff itself
represents the spinal column.
See also **chakra**

candida

A fungus which is a normal inhabitant of the human gut and
often present in the mouth and vagina, since it particularly
likes to colonize warm and moist areas; also known as *monilia*
(*candida albicans*). If present in excessive amounts, it may
become invasive and cause disease. This can present as a
local infection, such as mucositis (*thrush*) or may also lead to

non-specific illness and various types of allergy, particularly to foodstuffs. This happens especially in immuno-suppressed people including babies, the elderly, diabetics, and patients taking antibiotic or steroid treatment for other types of illness.

carnelian

A pink, red, or brown stone which is said to strengthen courage and ambition. It is particularly used on the spleen chakra (**manipura**), where it is believed to be good for the blood and also to help with digestive problems.
See also **crystal therapy**

cellular regeneration

A therapy designed with the object of regenerating the body on a cellular level. It uses a variety of techniques, including conscious thought, diet and dietary supplements, breathing exercises, and meditation.

cellular therapy

See **live cell therapy**

cellulite

A type of fatty tissue, claimed to be distinctive by some 'beauty experts', the presence of which is linked to hormone changes particularly associated with the female menopause. There is no orthodox evidence that cellulite is any different from any other type of fat, but there is a distinct distribution, with fatty accumulations on thighs, buttocks, upper arms, and abdomen with a characteristic lumpy and dimpled appearance. Naturopaths believe that this results from the western style of diet, with an excess of starch, fat protein, and sugar, and that some improvement may occur with dietary treatment, exercise, and skin brushing.

centaury /ˈsɛntɔːri/

A **Bach flower remedy** said to help people who are easily taken advantage of, or who have difficulty in standing up for themselves.

cerato /səˈrɑːtoʊ/
A **Bach flower remedy** said to help people who have no confidence in their own judgement, are easily influenced by other people's opinions, and are in constant need of reassurance from others.

chakra
One of the energy centres of the yogic system, which roughly correspond to plexuses of the autonomic nervous system. They are visualized as vortices in the body's energy fields which are important in channelling consciousness and linking the physical and spiritual dimensions. There are seven chakras:

base chakra see **muladhara**;
abdominal chakra see **swadhistana**;
solar plexus chakra see **manipura**;
heart chakra see **anahata**;
throat chakra see **vishuddi**;
command chakra see **ajna**;
crown chakra see **sahasra**.

channelling
A process in which a healer acts as a route, or channel, through which an external energy source can flow. The term usually applies to the channelling of healing energies which can then be directed to the patient to produce beneficial effects. This may involve the intervention of spirits or of God (for spiritual healers), and may also be used to communicate ideas and messages from some external intelligent sources which some believe to be of divine or extraterrestrial origin.

charismatic healing
[Greek *charis* 'grace'] A form of divine healing based on the Christian faith and, in particular, on the power of personal prayer for the blessing of good health. It aims both to prevent sickness and to release healing forces to those suffering from disease processes.

cheirology /kaɪˈrɒlədʒi/
The art of hand analysis, which interprets the personality, character, and temperament from the shape and the lines of the hand. Some practitioners combine the principles of **TCM** and the **five elements** with modern psychology, which may allow a more detailed assessment of emotional and sexual problems as well as the individual's creative potential.

chelation therapy /kəˈleɪʃn/
A biochemical treatment in which a mixture of minerals, vitamins, and enzymes is given intravenously to bind and remove heavy metals and calcium. This is an orthodox treatment for heavy metal poisoning, but its effects are not well substantiated when applied to patients with heart problems in order to remove calcium deposits from arterial walls and to unblock blood vessels without the need for operation.
See also **EDTA**

cherry plum
A deciduous shrub (*Prunus cerasifera*) with white flowers, also known as *myrobalan*, from which a **Bach flower remedy** can be prepared. This is said to help those who lack emotional control, are subject to irrational outbursts, are in a desperate frame of mind, or suffer from a fear of insanity.

chestnut bud
A **Bach flower remedy** which is said to help those who continually repeat the same mistakes and are unable to learn from their experience.

chi
See **qi**

chicory
A **Bach flower remedy** for those who have a mothering disposition, being possessive and overprotective, and who attempt to hold on to their loved ones.

chi kung
See qi gong

chiropody
The study of the structure and function of the foot, and of therapy dedicated to the prevention and treatment of foot disorders; also known as *podiatry*, especially in American English. It now extends to the treatment of sport and dance injuries of the feet.

chiropractic
[Greek *cheir* 'hand' + *praktikos* 'done by'] The study of health and disease from a structural point of view, with special emphasis on spinal mechanics and its effect on the nervous system. The discipline was founded in 1895 by Daniel David Palmer (1845–1913), a 'magnetic healer' who founded the Palmer School of Chiropractic in 1895, which is probably now the most widely recognized alternative medical practice in the Western world. The fundamental concept is that small misalignments (*subluxations*) of the spine can cause neurological defects and muscular and skeletal dysfunction, which leads to pain and also diseases of internal organ systems. Examination by a practitioner may include the use of X-rays and blood tests, and treatment is entirely by **manipulation** directed at the spinal column, usually consisting of short, forceful thrusting movements to restore the normal alignment of spine and pelvis.

chlorella
An edible green freshwater plant cultivated in China. It is exceptionally rich in many micronutrients, including calcium, iron, trace elements such as zinc and selenium, vitamins A, B complex, C, and E.

Christian Scientists
A Christian sect founded in 1879 as the First Church of Christ, Scientist, in Boston USA by Mary Baker Eddy (1821–1910) who believed that healing is proof of God's love, and that drawing close to God and living according to the principles of divine harmony are prerequisites in all healing

processes. Although consulting conventional doctors is not forbidden in the sect, many of its members prefer to pray and trust in God even when suffering severe illnesses. American life insurance companies give them preferential rates because they are such a good health risk.

chromotherapy
The use of the three primary colours (red, green, violet) for healing purposes.
See also **colour therapy**

chronic fatigue syndrome
See **myalgic encephalomyelitis**

chronobiology
The study of **biorhythms** and their effects. It makes extensive use of computer techniques to construct charts of the interacting cycles.

chrysolite
See **peridot**

citrine
A type of quartz associated with the sun, which is said to open up a bridge between the lower (logical) and the higher (intuitive) mind. This encourages clear thinking, receptivity, decisiveness, and communicative skills.
See also **crystal therapy**

clairvoyance
One of the three main categories of extra-sensory perception, referring to the possession of a psychic gift which may be a useful adjunct to conventional techniques of diagnosis for both physical and psychological disease. Particular diseases may have *auric profiles* which can be read by the clairvoyant directly without recourse to any conventional diagnostic techniques.

clematis

A woody climbing plant with tendrils and brightly coloured flowers from which a **Bach flower remedy** can be prepared. It is said to help those people who live in a dream-world of their own and who are inattentive and absent-minded. They often see themselves as creative and artistic, but require assistance to cope effectively with everyday life.

client-centred therapy

See **Rogerian counselling**

clinical ecology

A study of the effect of the environment on health. Ecological illnesses may be either recognized clinical entities which clearly have an ecological basis, or non-specific diseases whose underlying cause may be wholly or partly ecological. The pathology of these illnesses is mostly blamed on food allergy and chemical sensitivity. The symptoms tend to be non-specific, and a scoring system has been devised such that if any five of the nine symptoms listed below are present, then the problem is likely to have a clinical ecology component.

1 excessive fatigue and general malaise;
2 abdominal distention with flatulence and diarrhoea, frequently worse after eating;
3 headaches and migraine;
4 fluctuations in weight;
5 lack of concentration, forgetfulness, anxiety, and depression; called *brain fog* by American clinical ecologists;
6 excessive sweating, particularly at night;
7 palpitations with no obvious cause;
8 rheumatic aches and pains;
9 insomnia.

Investigation may include **cytotoxic testing,** a **sublingual drop test, kinesiology,** or a **radio-allergic solvents test**. Treatment often includes an **elimination diet.**

co-counselling

A system introduced from the USA in the 1970s in which people who desire self-development are paired together and take it in turns to act as counsellor or client to each other. There is a short training course before they practise together in this way for their mutual benefit.

co-enzyme Q10

A naturally occurring constituent of mitochondria, where it plays an essential part in releasing energy from food. Q10 supplements are recommended for the elderly, and for those with active lifestyles (eg sportsmen/women) who require an energy boost.

cognitive psychotherapy

A form of psychotherapy introduced in the 1960s by American psychologist Aaron Beck which teaches people to think and act in a positive rather than a negative way. It is believed that behaviour is conditioned by previous experiences which have resulted in the adoption of particular views and assumptions, so that people perceive themselves in a particular way. This can affect their feelings and emotions and the way in which they process information, ie the way they behave and solve problems. It is possible to make a conscious decision to change these assumptions and viewpoints with the aim of boosting the self-confidence of those with a poor self-image, which will then result in a change of their behaviour.

colon cleansing

A technique which has the aim of keeping the colon clean and functioning properly to maintain good health. This is usually accomplished by eating natural vegetable fibres to eliminate waste from the body and to assist with the absorption of nutrients from the diet. Various herbal mixtures are also available which are claimed to condition the whole intestine. See also **colonic irrigation**

colonic irrigation

A technique in which water is pumped into the colon so as to cleanse it and remove toxic waste. This procedure may be used in preparation for bowel surgery but also as a treatment for bowel dysfunction, and is incidentally said to improve the condition of both skin and hair.

See also **colon cleansing**

colour breathing

A form of **meditation** which is best practised either in the early morning or on retiring at night, in which the subject is aware of the colours pouring in from the natural sunlight or light from a treatment lamp and concentrates on enjoying the exhilarating and beneficial effects of this radiation. Some-times a **mantra** is chanted which is attuned to the colour being used, and lights of particular colours may be used to treat specific problems. Red light is claimed to benefit paralysis in both adults and children. Orange light has been used to treat cholera as well as gall stones and kidney stones. Yellow is helpful for diabetes and constipation. Green is used for ulcers, colds, flu, and breast cancer. Blue is for fever, inflammation, dysentery, teething, cuts, and burns.

colour therapy

The use of coloured light for healing, a practice which dates back to ancient Greece and the Healing Temples of Light and Colour at Heliopolis in Egypt. Energy and radiation affect living cells, and since both infra-red and ultra-violet radiation are known to have healing properties, so visible light may also produce healing, and this may not be dependent upon actually seeing the colour. Colour therapists may be able to tell, by looking at a subject, what colour they are deficient in, or may use a **Kilner screen** to view a patient's **aura**. The medical history and horoscope may be consulted before specific colours are chosen, and various wavelengths are thought to energize specific organs and tissues. The psychological and physical effects of coloured light are well researched; for example, red light has been shown to consistently raise blood pressure, whereas blue light has a calming effect. The selection of colours for home decoration, and for clinics andwork-places, may have significant effects upon the occupants. A colour therapist, as well as using coloured light, may also advise on clothing and diet so that, for example, a patient deficient in the colour red may be advised to eat beetroot, radishes, and red fruits.

See also **rainbow healing**

complementary medicine

A general term encompassing those therapies which can be used as an adjunct to conventional Western allopathic medicine. They are not intended to provide an alternative to orthodox treatment.

See also **alternative medicine**

compress

A cloth or towel soaked in hot or cold water, wrung out, and applied to whichever part of the body requires treatment. Hot compresses increase the blood flow through the area, promote sweating, and so flush out any obstruction or toxins that are present. Cold compresses cause constriction of the blood vessels and reduce the blood flow through the area, which may thus reduce swelling and inflammation.

conditioning

A learning process described by Russian psychologist Ivan Pavlov (1849–1936), who trained dogs to salivate when a bell was rung by associating the sound of the bell with their feeding time. He described this learned behaviour as a 'conditioned reflex'.

See also **behaviour therapy**

copper bracelet

A traditional way of treating arthritis and rheumatism. It may be that trace quantities of copper are absorbed through the skin in sufficient quantities to offset tissue copper deficiency. Three-quarters of patients claim some relief of symptoms using such bracelets.

coral

A natural rock-like substance formed from the skeletons of marine polyps, found as reefs in warm, shallow seas. It is found in a variety of colours including white, red, and brown. It is recommended as a balancing stone for those working in the caring professions, and is said to protect against negative attitudes and to support physical work.

See also **crystal therapy**

corona discharge

An electrical discharge which occurs in an intense electric field resulting in the emission of blue light. A photograph of the aura (*corona*) associated with an object can be taken by exposing film directly to high voltage, high frequency electric discharge passing from the object through the film to a conducting plate. This process was originally described by Yakub O Yodko-Narkevitch in 1850.

See also **Kirlian photography**

Couéism /ˈkuːeɪzm/

A technique based on the views of the French apothecary Emile Coué (1857–1926), who developed the catch-phrase 'every day, in every way, I am getting better and better'. He believed that, with repetition, this phrase would enter the mind and have a beneficial influence on unconscious processes.

See also **autosuggestion**

counselling

A term covering a wide variety of techniques of consultation and dispensing information and advice according to the various interests, training, and experience of a therapist or counsellor. Advice is generally given on specific topics or problems, such as sexual behaviour or financial difficulties, but may also include psychotherapeutic techniques or body therapies.

crab apple

A **Bach flower remedy** to help put things in perspective and to cleanse the body or mind. It may be useful after suffering a disease or for those who feel themselves polluted in some way.

cranial osteopathy

A technique of manipulating the bones of the skull using light pressure of the hands. It was developed in the USA by William Garner Sutherland in the 1920s. Examination allows the practitioner to detect and correct pressure and distortion in the skull and facial bones using gentle manipulation, and while pressure is applied by the hands the practitioner visualizes the skull bones as moving freely at their points of contact. The beneficial effects are sometimes said to result from influencing the energy field rather than the actual bones themselves. The technique is said to be useful for sufferers from migraine and other forms of headache, as well as for those with persistent discomfort following head injury or whiplash.

cranial rhythm impulse (CRI)

A palpable rhythmic pulsation around the head and body with a normal frequency of 6–12 cycles per minute, which is not related to other body rhythms such as breathing or heart rate. It is said to be due to the cumulative effects of pressure changes in the cerebro-spinal fluid (CSF) which result from changes in both the breathing rate and depth of breathing. The arterial pulse acts as a force factor in 'mixing' the CSF, but otherwise does not affect the impulse itself.

See also **cranio-sacral therapy**

cranio-sacral therapy (CST)

A form of manipulation which is said to release the tensions and imbalances in the cranial rhythm, a movement arising in the membranes and bones of the skull and transmitted throughout the body via the connective tissues. The skull and the brain within are thought to expand and contract, and the flow of cerebrospinal fluid may be affected by the anatomical-relationships between the brain, meninges, and cranialbones. **CST** involves gentle manipulation, focusing on themembranes as the source of cranio-sacral dysfunction to restore the free movement which is necessary for the health of the central nervous system and to release blockages which may result in emotional or physical dysfunction. The technique may be applied to a wide variety of disorders, including physical injuries, functional and emotional disorders, chronic neck and back pains, and the symptoms following traumatic head injury.

See also **cranial rhythm impulse**

CRI

See **cranial rhythm impulse**

cryotherapy

The use of cold to reduce inflammation and swelling. The application of cold in the form of ice or cryogel causes initial vasoconstriction, but this is followed by a reflex vasodilation which increases capillary blood flow to the tissues and reduces oedema. The technique is used by osteopaths, chiropractors, and physiotherapists, and may include the application of cold sprays to myofascial **trigger points**.

crystal

A stone said to generate energy and repel negativity. It can open up higher levels of awareness and remove stagnation in life, thoughts, and attitudes. It has been claimed to help with heart, spine, and hearing difficulties.

See also **crystal therapy**

crystal therapy

A type of therapy using crystals (which include precious and semi-precious stones), thought to generate healing vibrations which may act upon the body's energy field. They are said to increase available energy and correct energy imbalance and

blockages. The use of a crystal may increase awareness of the body's own circulating energies and promote the healing of physical or emotional problems. Crystals can be used to channel healing energies from a healer to a patient. They may be placed on specific parts of the body requiring treatment, including acupuncture points.
See also **crystal; fluorite**

CST
See **cranio-sacral therapy**

cun /sʊn/
A Chinese unit of measurement which is used to locate acupuncture points by referring to the patient's own personal scaling system. One cun is the length of the middle phalanx of the middle finger or the width of the interphalangeal joint of the thumb. The width of the hand at the proximal interphalangeal joint is 3 cun. The arm from elbow to wrist measures 12 cun. The leg from knee to ankle measures 16 cun.
See also **traditional Chinese medicine**

cupping
An ancient technique in which a vacuum is created inside a jar or cup, using a burning taper or swab. The cup is then applied to specific points on the body, usually acupuncture points, to disperse congestion. The technique is popular for treating sprains, arthritis, and bronchitis, and sometimes medicinal herbs are placed inside the cup. The partial vacuum draws flesh up into the cup which thus becomes attached. The skin becomes red because of an increased blood flow through it and there is occasional bruising of delicate skin. According to **traditional Chinese medicine**, cupping draws perverse energy to the surface and disperses it.

cymatics /saɪˈmætɪks/
[Greek *kyma* 'a great wave'] A form of **sound therapy**, developed in the 1960s by British physician Peter Manners, in which high frequency sound waves are directed at specific

affected areas of the body in order to retune any disharmony. Treatment may be given in a treatment pool with a background of relaxing music. Good results have been reported in relieving arthritis, rheumatism, and back pains. There is some evidence that post-operative wound healing may be accelerated.

cytotoxic testing

A form of **allergy** testing. A blood sample is taken from which white blood cells are separated and exposed to concentrates of various foods and chemicals. These may be observed to undergo changes if the patient is allergic to the provoking substance. Unfortunately this is a very subjective test which is difficult to interpret.

D

dance therapy

A form of therapy, introduced in the USA in the 1940s, and developed by Gabrielle Roth in the late 1970s, which encourages spontaneous movements rather than formal dance sequences. It is usually practised as a form of **group therapy** and, when practised regularly, helps to rid the body of tension and rigidity and develop movement from the centre. This may be especially useful for people who have difficulty in talking about their feelings, as it can allow them to make contact with the contents of their unconscious mind. Dance therapy is also used to improve mobility in patients who have nervous and muscular disorders, such as those recovering from strokes, and it is recommended for the elderly to keep their joints and spines supple, as well as providing a meeting-point for people who would otherwise be isolated. The relationship between body, movement, and emotions can help to express feelings which are not easily put into words. This non-verbal form of psychotherapy can give psychological and emotional support to those who might not be receptive to other techniques, such as people with learning difficulties.

decoction

[Latin *decoquere* 'to boil down'] A herbal drink prepared by adding boiling water to powdered dried herbs or roots, and then simmering for 10 or 15 minutes to produce a 'tea'. This procedure extracts the water-soluble parts of the substance, allowing the insoluble constituents to be strained or filtered out.

diagnosis

A statement of the nature of a patient's disease, or the process by which a practitioner (whether orthodox or conventional) interprets the nature of the problem. This usually involves taking a history of the problem, performing some sort of physical examination, and then possibly conducting tests, the nature of which will depend upon the background and training of the practitioner. Making a diagnosis allows the practitioner to understand the cause (*aetiology*) and mechanism of an illness, and then to formulate an appropriate treatment.

diamond

A form of crystalline carbon produced by high temperature and pressure in the earth's crust; the hardest natural substance known. It is highly valued as a gemstone, and symbolizes durability, hardness, and incorruptibility. It is said to stimulate clear mental vision, prevent dreaming, and to dispel negativity.

doctrine of signatures

The teaching, which may have been popularized by Paracelsus (1493–1541), that God created plants in certain shapes so that men would know which plants to use for treating which illnesses. If a plant or part of a plant looks like a body organ then it may contain healing properties related to that organ so that a remedy can be prepared from it. Examples include *hepatica* for liver ailments and *wood sorrel* for heart trouble.

dogmatic therapeutics

One of two basic approaches to medical treatment expounded in Classical Roman and Greek medical texts.

The dogmatic approach requires a knowledge of the cause of the disease so that the therapy can be decided upon rationally. If it has been correctly deduced, then the therapy is bound to work, and so does not need to be validated by subsequent observation.
See also **empirical therapeutics**

do-in /ˈdoʊ ˈɪn/

[Japanese, 'self stimulation'] A form of **acupressure** massage, originating in China in c.2600 BC, which is applied to oneself, either to specific areas that require massage or systematically working along the **acupuncture meridians**. It can be applied both for treatment and also to prevent disease by balancing the body's energy.

douching /ˈduːʃɪŋ/
A form of **hydrotherapy** in which jets of water are directed on to various parts of the body, using a range of water pressures and temperatures. The process is said to stimulate the circulation, and to ease muscular and other pains including lumbago and rheumatism.

dowsing
[Cornish, 'striking'] A process in which a rod or other indicator moves or vibrates in the hands of a person as he or she approaches a particular substance in the ground. Dowsing has been used to search for water, oil, and mineral deposits, and also to locate missing objects including archaeological remains. There are agricultural and horticultural uses, and it has also been employed in selecting sites for building. The first recorded use is in ancient Egypt, and the first mention in English literature is 1240; but its use for medical purposes dates from the 1920s, when the French priest Abbé Mermet used a dowsing technique (with a pendulum) to locate and diagnose diseased organs. A pendulum may be used to select homeopathic remedies. The procedure always requires a human being as an intermediary, and so has been described as a 'supersensory' phenomenon, since the dowser is thought to detect and then amplify whatever radiations may be emanating from the substance being dowsed.

dysbiosis
A term describing colonic dysfunction which is due to a disturbance in the numbers and proportions of the bacteria living in the gut (the gut flora). It was suggested that at one time or another up to 50% of the population show an alteration in the balance of their normal gut flora. If the integrity of the lining of the gut (the mucosa) is disturbed, then the gut may absorb active peptides which can produce a wide range of symptoms.

Treatment can be by a naturopathic diet approach to allow the patient to regain a normal food tolerance, and this may be assisted with homeopathic preparations. It may also be useful to recolonize the gut with 'friendly' bacteria.

See also **clinical ecology; naturopathy; probiotics**

dzogchen

A meditation system in the ancient traditions of Tibetan Buddhism.

The technique emphasizes a simple, direct-access, 'self-liberated' state, without the use of a **mantra, visualization**, or other methods.

E

ear acupuncture
See **auricular therapy**

ear candles
A form of candle, originally used by the Hopi Indians, and now widely adopted in Europe. The candles are hollow and lined with silver foil. They are inserted into the ear orifice, and when ignited produce local heat which stimulates the circulation and local energy points. As the candles burn they exert a mild suction, and vapour from the herbal extracts contained in the candles is circulated into the external ear. The herbs include sage and camomile, which may themselves have soothing properties. This is an effective way of softening and extracting ear wax.

earth medicine
A group of therapies based on the worship of the Earth Mother or Goddess, encompassing knowledge of witchcraft, **mineral therapy, crystal therapy**, and flower remedies. This knowledge is said to be derived from 'ancient wisdom', and is passed amongst women healers working in the spirit of the Earth Mother.
See also **Bach flower remedies**

eclosion system
A computer system developed by Dr William Nelson in the 1980s which incorporates special attachments allowing measurements and recordings of clinical importance such as temperature, skin resistance, ECG, EEG, EMG, and gastric motility. Further information from other sources, such as blood, urine, or hair analysis results, and details of personal and medical history, can also be fed into the system and the data then analysed to produce a differential diagnosis and

treatment recommendations. The system is programmed to recommend alternative or natural therapies and remedies, including an assessment of nutritional requirements. There is a **biofeedback** facility which can feed such data as voltage, current, resistance, and temperature back to the operator to allow self-monitoring and regulation.

eco diseases

A group of health problems caused by environmental pollution, either directly by exposure to an environmental hazard (eg in an industrial setting) or indirectly by general exposure to toxins and pollutants in the air, water, and food supplies (eg lead and pesticides).

ecology

See **clinical ecology**

EDTA

An abbreviation of **e**thylene **d**iamine **t**etra-**a**cetic acid. This is a widely-used chelating agent (see **chelation therapy**) which combines with heavy metals or other toxic minerals, but also with essential metals such as iron, zinc, and magnesium causing unwanted toxic effects. EDTA may be given orally or intravenously, and similar substances are found in some natural foods including baked beans, seaweed, bananas, and eggs.

electrical skin resistance (ESR)

A characteristic of the skin which can be monitored with a meter and which changes according to the local blood flow in the skin. This is influenced by autonomic nervous system (ANS) activity which controls the amount of sweating. The ESR thus gives a measure of the activity of the sweat glands on the palms of the hands and the soles of the feet which indirectly indicates ANS activity and relaxation. The principle forms the basis of many *relaxation meters*.
See also **biofeedback; galvanic skin response**

electro-acupuncture

A technique developed by the Chinese in the 1950s which has, to a large extent, replaced manual stimulation of acupuncture needles. The acupuncture needles are inserted into the relevant points, and pulsed electrical current is then passed between pairs of needles. The frequency and amplitude of the current can be varied according to the effects desired, but generally a low frequency stimulus (2–10Hz) has been shown to cause release of endogenous opiates, and a high frequency stimulus (500–1000Hz) blocks the transmission of pain impulses and is used for acupuncture anaesthesia.

See also **electrotherapy; endorphins**

electromagnetic smog

A generic term for the environmental stress produced by many varieties of **electro-pollution**.

See also **resonance therapy**

electro-pollution

A term used for the ill effects caused by high and low frequency electromagnetic emissions (**EMF**) resulting from increased domestic and commercial use of electricity (eg from microwaves, high voltage cables, and computer terminals). There may be adverse long-term effects from this radiation, which leads to nausea, headaches, impaired concentration, stress, and possibly even cancer. Specialist advice is now available on the biological effects of electromagnetism, and steps can be taken to protect against the unwanted effects of EMF at home and at work.

See also **air imbalance**

electrotherapy

A technique which involves discharging electric currents through the skin and underlying tissues for the relief of pain and acceleration of healing. A variety of devices is available.

See also **electro-acupuncture; TENS**

eleutherococcus senticosus /elju:θərouˈkɒkəs sentɪˈkousəs/

A thorny shrub of the family *Araliaceae*, which is related to **ginseng** and which grows in Siberia and China. It is used as a tonic to increase energy and resistance to disease, and acts as an **adaptogen** by assisting the body's own natural defences. Many Chinese believe that regular use increases longevity and may help to restore memory. It is used by some athletes to improve their stamina. The active constituents are called *eleutherosides* (A to E), and the pharmacology of these substances is being investigated at Moscow State University and the University of Munich. Many clinical studies were organized in the USSR, particularly in the fields of oncology and cardiovascular disease.

ELFs

An abbreviation of **E**xtremely **L**ow **F**requency electromagnetic waves, which are emitted from electrical equipment (including radios, televisions and computers). Various studies suggest that there may be damaging effects from these emissions. Russian research links ELFs with nervous system disorders, hormone changes, and chromosome damage, and a Norwegian study has shown a two-fold increase in the development of cancer of the breast in male workers exposed to ELF electromagnetic fields.

elimination diet

A method of **allergy** testing developed by Dr Albert Rowe in the 1920s, in which particular kinds of food are omitted from the diet (eg grains or dairy food) and the effect on the patient's symptoms is assessed. Elimination of one or several foods may relieve various symptoms such as headaches, rheumatism, or an irritable bowel, and foods may then be reintroduced one by one to identify the provoking agents. Testing in this way is more effective after preliminary fasting and detoxification to put the patient into a hypersensitive state. Foods that most commonly cause sensitivity reactions are milk and dairy products, wheat, coffee, chocolate, eggs, and citrus fruits.

elm

A deciduous tree (*Ulmus procera*) with tiny flowers from which a **Bach flower remedy** can be prepared. It is recommended for those who lack confidence, who are worried at their ability to cope, and who feel overwhelmed by their responsibilities.

emerald

A variety of beryl, the commercial ore of beryllium, in the form of a green gemstone. It is related to the heart **chakra**, and is known as the 'stone of Venus' since it is said to promote love. It has been used as a panacea for promoting peace and relaxation, soothing pain and inflammation, stimulating brain and memory, and developing clairvoyance.
See also **crystal therapy**

emotional rhythm

A **biorhythm** reflected in a person's mood, cheerfulness, sensitivity, and creativity, related to the functioning of the nervous and endocrine systems. The **biorhythms** follow alternative positive and negative phases, so that when the emotional balance is in a positive phase people are cheerful and optimistic, but in a negative phase they are irritable, despondent, and depressed.

empirical (*or* empiric) therapeutics

One of two basic approaches to medical treatment expounded in Classical Roman and Greek medical texts. In following the empiric approach the patient's clinical symptoms lead the physician directly to some form of practical treatment, regardless of the theoretical considerations. The outcome of the treatment (ie success or failure) must then be assessed. The *empiric triad* which summarizes this approach consists of observation, comparison of the data with the literature, and conclusions drawn by analogy with previous similar circumstances.
See also **dogmatic therapeutics**

encounter groups

A form of **group therapy** developed by American psychologist Carl Rogers (1902–87) in the 1940s. Working in a group allows people to practise expressing their thoughts and feelings, and to share emotional experiences, in order to develop self-awareness and sensitivity towards others and thereby to improve social relationships.

endorphins

A family of naturally-occurring, opiate-like neuro-transmitters, identified and isolated in 1975 by the British neuroscientist John Hughes (1942–   ) and British pharmacologist Hans Walter Kosterlink (1903–   ); they are found in the brain and spinal cord and can be measured in the serum and cerebrospinal fluid. Electrical stimulation of some parts of the brain may cause massive increases in endorphin levels, and this may result in long-lasting pain relief. Both **electro-acupuncture** and **TENS** promote endorphin release in the central nervous system.

energetic herbalism

A recently developed system of therapy, pioneered by American herbalist and acupuncturist Michael Tietra. It combines the diagnostic principles of **traditional Chinese medicine** with the use of both Western and Chinese herbs for treatment.

energy cyst

A concept used in cranio-sacral **osteopathy** which may (or may not) have a physical reality. Injurious energies such as trauma or invading pathogens are thought to create a localized area of increased energy which becomes 'walled off' by the body. This energy cyst may create obstruction to the flow of **qi** through the **meridians**, causing pain, interference with local tissue function, and the development of **facilitated segments**.

energy medicine

An approach which takes concepts from modern physics and applies them to the electro-dynamic fields of the human body and their derangement in disease states. Orthodox medicine still largely holds a mechanistic view of body function, but many alternative therapies have a more dynamic approach to the body, and exploit concepts of energy flow in their diagnosis and treatment of illness.

enteropuncture

A technique using the **acupuncture** points distributed around the pyloric antrum of the stomach, which relate to the whole body in the same way as do points on the ears (see **auricular therapy**.)

Key points are present throughout the intestines and can be reached by endoscopy. Since perforation of the skin is not required at present, European law imposes no restrictions on who can perform this technique.

enzyme supplements
A way of helping people who suffer from long-standing digestive problems, sometimes accompanied by allergies. In some cases these may be contributed to by an enzyme deficiency. Various mixtures of digestive enzymes are available to be taken as an aid to digestion when used as a dietary supplement.

ESR
See **electrical skin resistance**

essential oils
Complex natural volatile oils which are extracted from plants and show chemical and medicinal properties. They are used in cosmetics, food, and toiletries, as well as in **aromatherapy**. Some oils have hormonal properties; for example sarsparilla has a testosterone-like action, and both hops and fennel contain oestrogen-like substances. Therapeutic actions documented include the anti-spasmodic effect of peppermint, the anti-hypertensive effect of calamus, and the expectorant action of lemon oil. The oils are mostly found in the leaves of the plant, where they form a barrier which helps to reduce water loss, but they may also be concentrated in other parts of the plant (eg lavender oil in the flowers, sandalwood in the bark, myrrh in the resin, and orange in the rind of the fruit).

eurhythmy
A concept based on the original ideas of Austrian social philosopher Rudolph Steiner (1861–1925), and developed by Swiss composer Emile Jacques-Dalcroze (1865–1951), in

which rhythmical movements are performed in harmony with the rhythm of the spoken word. The movements encourage rapid response to the changing rhythms, and seek to express gestures and postures which are inherent in speech and music. The approach can be used to develop self-expression, and as a form of therapy to correct habitual harmful movements and postures.

eye therapy
See **Bates' method**

F

facilitated segments

A concept in cranio-sacral **osteopathy** in which injury causes a local increase in the electrical conductivity of a tissue, and thus hypersensitivity and excitability of that segment of the spinal cord. There may be a resultant change in the texture of the tissue, and possibly local pain and tenderness.

faith healing

An approach based on the principle that whatever one truly believes can be made to happen and that, by bringing the sufferer into contact with supernatural forces, miraculous cures may be possible. Such techniques are usually practised within the context of an organized religion, using the power of God. Patients may also believe in the healing powers of objects and holy places; for example many pilgrims travel to Lourdes with faith in their chance of a cure, even though they know that the statistical chance of a cure is small.
See also **spiritual healing**

family therapy

A form of psychiatric treatment developed in the 1960s for families in difficulty, conducted by specially-trained family therapists. Problems may include difficulties in relationships between family members, such as those of adolescence, divorce, and bereavement. The therapists will generally guide the family unit to find its own best solution by discussion and agreement between its members, rather than attempting to impose an external solution.

Feldenkrais method /'feldnkraɪs/

A system of slow exercises designed to eliminate habitual acquired restrictive movement patterns and postures and to regain free body movements. It was devised by Moshe

Feldenkrais, a Jewish nuclear physicist who escaped to England from Nazi-occupied France during World War II. He believed that new patterns could be established in the brain so that movements would be made more efficiently, and that by changing these harmful physical patterns the mental and emotional states would also benefit. The two aspects of practice are **awareness through movement**, conducted as class sessions, and **functional integration**, conducted as individual sessions where the teacher will physically guide the pupil's body through the correct movements.

feng shui

[Chinese, 'under the canopy of heaven'] A discipline originally used to divine the most auspicious site to place a tomb, where the ancestor's spirit could be in harmony with heaven and earth. This was later extended to advice on the positioning of buildings, and it is even possible to incorporate the principles of the Taoist text, the *I Ching*, into the architecture itself. The objective is to achieve harmony with nature by positioning objects and structures such as buildings, rooms, furniture, and gardens to be in sympathy with the flow of the earth's energy. Practitioners search for lines of **qi** in the environment, and use these lines to enhance the balance of nature in the area for the benefit of the people there, who should then enjoy increased prosperity, good health, and happiness.
See also **geomancy**

fibre

A dietary constituent required as *roughage*, since it is not digested or absorbed but remains inside the bowel giving bulk to the faeces and stimulating bowel movement. It consists mainly of cellulose which is found in plant cells, especially in roots, stems, and seed coats, but also includes lignin from woody plants and pectins found in fruits. Fibre is said to reduce the incidence of constipation, haemorrhoids and cancer of the bowel, as well as having a beneficial effect on other bowel and cardiovascular problems.

five elements

The basic elements of **traditional Chinese medicine**: wood, fire, earth, metal and water. These are portrayed as a constantly turning circle which allows the student to visualize the interchange and interrelationships between the elements. The elements are associated with the internal organs, senses, emotions, colours, foods, and other phenomena, which can thereby be classified using this system. The interactions are shown in the **sheng** (generating), **ko** (controlling), and **wu** (counteracting) **cycles**.

flooding

A technique of **behaviour therapy** in which the patient's fears and phobias can be treated by directly confronting them with the objects or situations of which they are afraid; also known as *forced exposure*. Although they may be initially terrified, the fear should gradually subside and allow them to place the object of their fears in perspective, resulting in a return to rational behaviour.

flotation therapy

A therapy devised by American psychoanalyst and neuro-physiologist Dr John C Lily, who believed that the brain could focus better on its own internal mental processes if not distracted by external stimuli. External stimuli, including gravity, can be minimized by floating in a closed tank of warm water to which a high concentration of Epsom Salts has been added to increase buoyancy. The water is usually c.25 cm deep and at a temperature of 34.2°C, and the tank in total or semi-darkness in a light and sound-proofed room. The buoyancy gives a weightless feeling, and the aim of the treatment is total relaxation of mind and body and the release of stress. Flotation is said to eliminate harmful chemicals and toxins, to be good for stiffness and structural or muscular problems, and to counteract anxiety, stress, and tension.

flower essences

Essences derived from flower petals. The petals have absorbed the sun's energy, and this, it is claimed, can be extracted by immersion in water and then bottled. The essences from particular flowers have specific actions when taken by mouth, and are claimed to help relieve anxiety, depression, and nervous disorders, and to encourage the expression of emotions and the harmonizing of mind, body, and spirit.

fluorite

A common mineral, calcium fluoride, in the form of a crystal said to represent the Holy Trinity, manifested in the purple, white, and green colours of the stone. It is claimed to be good for the bones and teeth, but also helps with the synthesis of ideas and the development of spiritual knowledge and awareness.

See also **crystal therapy**

focusing

A technique in which the mind is directed to developing an awareness of the body's inner self by paying attention to the body's own wisdom rather than by trying to resolve problems intellectually. This skill enhances other psychological processes such as exploring feelings and emotions, making choices and decisions, psychotherapy, self-help, and meditation.

folk healing

A term which encompasses a wide variety of techniques and traditions. Therapists using these methods are usually unlicensed practitioners without formal qualifications employing methods of treatment indigenous to the local population. Modern forms of folk healing in our present society might include **polarity therapy** and **sex therapy**.

food allergy

A true allergic reaction in which there is evidence of an abnormal immunological response to a food item. With a true **allergy** there is a reaction between the complement (a group of plasma components which help the reaction between an antigen and an antibody) and a type of immunoglobin (IgM or IgG), which results in kinin release and inflammation. Circulating immune complexes may be present after food

ingestion, and the condition is easily diagnosed by conventional skin testing and immunoglobin estimations (eg raised IgE).
See also **food sensitivity**

food sensitivity

A state in which, although there is an intolerance to certain food items, there is no evidence of an abnormal immunological reaction. Most food sensitivities are temporary, and consumption of the foods can be recommenced after a period of abstinence. If the subject can never tolerate the food item, the sensitivity is said to be *fixed*. The mechanisms involved in food sensitivity include enzyme deficiencies (eg lactase deficiency), psychological reactions to food, pharmacological reactions to food or food additives, food reactions which are caused by histamine release in sensitized individuals (eg shellfish or strawberry sensitivity), or a direct irritant effect of the food on the gut mucosa (eg wheat, bran, or spicy foods).
See also **food allergy**

forced exposure

See **flooding**

free radicals

Highly reactive, unstable molecules which have usually lost an electron, resulting in a chemical impetus to replace it (eg superoxide, hydroxyl radical, and singlet oxygen). They can be generated by body metabolism (eg liposomal enzymes in leucocytes) or from external sources (eg ozone, nuclear radiation, and environmental pollution).
See also **antioxidants**

fu

In **traditional Chinese medicine**, the hollow organs governed by the **yang** or positive forces: the stomach, large intestine, bladder, **triple heater**, gall bladder, and small intestine.
See also **yang; zang**

functional integration

An aspect of the **Feldenkrais method** in which the teacher uses manipulation to guide a pupil's body through a sequence of movements and postures designed to retrain muscles that are injured or dysfunctional. The problem might arise through brain or spinal damage, or possibly just through habitual misuse.

G

galvanic skin response

A technique for monitoring **electrical skin resistance**, but which uses a more sensitive meter that can detect much smaller changes in skin resistance. This type of apparatus is used as part of the lie detector machine, since it is sufficiently sensitive to identify emotional reactions in response to questioning.

galvanism

An early form of **electrotherapy** in which direct current was passed between skin electrodes placed on the surface of the body over areas of injury. It was used for treating sprains, strains, and sports injuries, particularly for pain relief. Galvanism was named after Italian physiologist Luigi Galvani (1739–98), who observed that a frog's leg would twitch if an electric current was applied to it.

garlic

A perennial bulb of the lily family (*Allium sativum*), used as a herbal remedy for at least 5000 years. It is available as oil, tablets, and fresh crushed cloves, and can be eaten, inhaled, or applied topically. It contains vitamins A, B_1, B_2, and C, and some natural antibiotics, anticoagulants, and cholesterol-lowering agents. The wide variety of uses includes treating bacterial and fungal infections, particularly of the gut, and possibly increasing resistance to viral infections such as colds, influenza, and herpes. Recently, German research has shown that garlic has a beneficial effect on natural killer (NK) cell activity in **AIDS** patients when it is eaten at doses of up to 10 grams daily.

See also **herbal medicine**

garnet

[Latin *granatus* 'like seeds'] A gemstone formed of silicates showing a wide range of colours but most commonly a deep red. In **crystal therapy** it is said to be good for male and female sexual problems, and is used to balance the base **chakra**. Garnet will also energize the circulation and encourage positive thinking.

gate control theory

A theory developed in 1965 which proposes that sensations felt by the body depend upon a balance of impulses travelling up the spinal cord along unmyelinated C fibres from peripheral receptors and myelinated A fibres which convey light touch. The two signals are integrated in the dorsal part of the spinal cord (the *substantia gelatinosa*), and stimulating A fibre activity can interfere with pain perception. This theory may explain the mechanism of **acupuncture** and **TENS**, which are thought to selectively stimulate A fibre activity, although other mechanisms such as the reticular activating system may also contribute.

gemstone therapy

Therapy based on the use of precious or semi-precious stones or minerals, which are thought to concentrate energy in their vibrations. These energies may help to relieve mental and emotional problems. In one form of therapy the vibrations from the gemstones are said to be transmitted to pure water by immersing the stones in water and leaving them in the sunshine. This creates an essence which may be absorbed by holding a bottle of energized water in the hand for several minutes and then placing drops from the bottle underneath the tongue.

See also **crystal therapy**

general adaptation syndrome

A description, developed by Hans Selye, of the reaction of a biological system (eg an animal) exposed to a hazardous environment. He described three stages:

Stage 1 the animal becomes hyperactive but non-adapted, e.g. in the presence of chronic physical irritant;

Stage 2 there is a stage of resistance and adaptation where the animal can tolerate the adverse condition;

Stage 3 the animal becomes exhausted and loses its ability to compensate, ie it reverts to being non-adapted.

gentian

A widely distributed perennial plant of the genus *Gentiana* sometimes used to prepare a **Bach flower remedy** recommended for people suffering discouragement and disappointment, and which is also helpful to those who lack confidence in themselves, especially after previous failures. It is said to encourage perseverance and discourage negative thinking.

geomancy

The study of 'earth mysteries' by detailed observation of the way in which the earth's energy affects daily life. Earth energy is said to flow through meridians known as ley lines which can be detected using a geomancer's compass, and this allows the geomancer to suggest the best position for a building and for the placement of design features such as doors and bedrooms to achieve the greatest harmony with nature and the environment. The word is also applied to divination by inspection of the lines and figures formed by scattering earth, or other material, on a surface.

See also **feng shui**

geopathic stress

Adverse effects resulting from electromagnetic fields and other forms of radiation from the earth. The consequences may result in insomnia, depression, hypertension, and even cancer. Environmental factors contributing to radiation which result in geopathic stress include **ley lines** and man-made structures such as power lines.

See also **geomancy; resonance therapy**

germanium

A metalloid element (atomic number 32) used as a semiconductor particularly in transistor manufacture, but also promoted as a stimulant for the immune system. It is non-essential as a nutrient, but has been claimed to have useful activity in AIDS patients and cancer sufferers. It was supplied as a non-toxic sesquioxide, but this may convert to toxic germanium dioxide on contact with stomach acid, and this raised doubts about its safety. It has now been withdrawn from use since it possibly causes kidney damage.

Gerson diet

A vegetarian diet developed in California by Dr Max Gerson in the 1920s to control his own migraine. The main feature is the daily intake of more than five pints of fresh raw juices, which include the juice of four pounds of raw organic carrots per day. The Gerson Clinic in Mexico offers an alternative approach to cancer treatment using this diet, following detoxification by coffee enemas, with additional nutritional supplements including high doses of vitamin C, large quantities of peppermint tea, and enzymes which are taken in the form of green leaf juice and fresh calf liver juice. The objectives are to strengthen the immune system so as to allow the body to fight the disease, to clear the body of toxins, to correct vitamin and mineral balance, and to encourage a positive attitude towards life. Although the cure rate is low, some patients report symptomatic improvement with reduced requirements for painkillers.

Gestalt therapy

[German *gestalt* 'whole, complete'] A technique of **psychotherapy**, developed by German psychoanalyst Fritz Perls (1893–1970) and his wife Laura in the 1960s, in which people are given responsibility for their thoughts and actions by making them aware of their own behaviour and by paying attention to non-verbal **body language**. Gestalt is symbolized by 'talking to the empty chair' — an unrehearsed imaginary conversation which may generate considerable emotion and provide the therapist with revealing insights into the patient's psyche. Gestalt is usually conducted as a **group therapy** in the form of short workshops (two or three days), during which time the participants are encouraged to behave in an expressive and spontaneous manner.

The underlying principle is that all aspects of the personality must respond to each external event, or inner conflict will result which distorts the behaviour pattern; each situation must be met with a complete response before moving on to, the next situation. The participants must be aware of their own thoughts, feelings, and actions, formulated in response to what is happening around them. The approach is particularly useful for those having difficulty expressing feelings and communicating with others, and for the treatment of tension and anxiety states.

gingko

A deciduous plant, originally from China, also known as the 'maiden hair tree' (*Gingko biloba*). It produces a seed with an edible kernel which contains active agents including glycosides, bioflavonoids, terpenes, and proanthocyanadins. These are said to improve the peripheral circulation, maintain the strength of capillary walls, inhibit platelet aggregation, increase cellular glucose uptake and energy production, and possibly influence neural transmission. The improved peripheral circulation may increase blood and oxygen supply to the brain, and for this reason gingko is recommended for use by the elderly. Some beneficial effects have been described in early Alzheimer's Disease.

ginseng

[Greek *panacea* 'all healing'] A perennial plant (*Panax ginseng*), cultivated in China, Korea, and Russia, whose powdered roots are renowned for having aphrodisiac properties, as well as being rejuvenating and useful as a tonic and dietary supplement. It contains saponin glycosides (or *ginsenosides*) that break down to produce sugars which may influence the immune system as well as increase resistance to infection, produce a mild anticoagulant effect on the blood, and protect tissues against damage caused by aging. Ginseng extract also contains a range of hormones and vitamins, and has been recommended for the treatment of headaches, tiredness, amnesia, and kidney, nervous, and circulatory problems.

gorse

A spiney shrub (*Ulex europaeus*) with yellow flowers from which a **Bach flower remedy** can be prepared for those with feelings of defeatism, pessimism and hopelessness.

graphology

The science of analysing handwriting as a guide to the character and personality of the writer. The study of handwriting dates back at least to the 16th century. A detailed analysis of the slant, shape, and depth of the letters, as well as of the general layout of the writing, enables the analyst to construct a picture of the character and personality of the writer, including their good and bad personality traits. This technique is now being used increasingly in industry to help assess a candidate's suitability for employment, and particularly to assess creative abilities and organizational skills. It has also proved valuable for forensic investigation.

green

In **colour therapy**, seen as the balance point between the 'hot' red colours and the 'cool' blue colours. It is the major healing colour of nature. Green is associated with the heart **chakra**, where it helps to develop a loving nature and to balance the analytical or intellectual side of the personality. Green persons are sensitive, responsive, and loving, but show a tendency to jealousy.

grounding

A notion used in **bioenergetics** which regards the legs and feet as being our contact with the realities of life (ie the ground or the earth). The way in which we stand and contact the earth (ie 'ground') is thus an expression of emotional balance. Exercises in grounding such as tiptoeing or stamping of the feet emphasize this connection.

group therapy

A form of psychotherapy, attributed to the American physician Joseph Hersey Pratt (1872–1942), which is conducted in small groups, and allows the individual to function in a social setting. It emphasizes the sharing of personal experiences and feelings, and is particularly useful for people with emotional difficulties and difficulties with social relationships. It can be valuable for group members to share their problems and learn from the experiences of others who have undergone similar difficulties. The support of such a group can help to overcome such problems as alcoholism and other forms of addiction.

See also **dance therapy; encounter groups; Gestalt therapy**

H

haematite
See **bloodstone**

hair diagnosis
The chemical analysis of a small hair sample to measure its mineral content. This can reveal nutritional imbalances and also detect harmful minerals which have been absorbed into the body, such as aluminium and lead. The results are very susceptible to sampling error, and the hair should preferably be taken from the nape of the neck (where it is quickest growing) and plucked out rather than cut. The part of the hair nearest the skin surface gives the most reliable sample, since the other end is more influenced by shampoos, sprays, and environmental contamination.

hakim
[Arabic, 'learned wise'] A term applied to judges, rulers, or governors in Muslim countries, but in the context of alternative medicine usually referring to Indian or Muslim herbal therapists who employ ready-prepared mixtures rather than making individual formulations for their patients.

hallucinogen
A drug that produces hallucinations. Of such drugs, *psychedelic* drugs (eg LSD) typically produce swirling arrays of strong colours and *psychomimetic* drugs act on the central nervous system, imitating aspects of natural regulatory activity (eg stimulation, sedation).

There are many naturally-occurring hallucinogens (eg 'magic mushrooms' and mescaline) which have been used for medical and religious purposes. These distort perception, and may lead the participants to believe that they have witnessed supernatural events or received divine revelations.

harmaline

A **hallucinogen**, extracted from a vine, which is used by Amazonian Indian shamans for healing, clairvoyance, and divination. It is structurally very similar to the beta-carbolines which are secreted by the **pineal gland**, and may be one of the chemical triggers for dreaming.
See also **shamanism**

harmonic technique

A type of osteopathic manipulation in which the practitioner causes different body masses to oscillate in accordance with the resonance of the tissues. This has a direct mechanical effect by stretching and compressing the tissue and stimulating blood circulation; but it also affects reflex activities such as relaxation, muscle spindle activity, and pain reflexes.
See also **osteopathy**

HARP

An abbreviation which is the code name for the *Healing **AIDS** Research Project* being conducted at the Bastyr College Research Department in Seattle, Washington, to study the effect of various complementary medical treatments on AIDS patients. The natural therapies studied include nutrition supplements, **herbal medicine** and **homeopathy, hydrotherapy, psychotherapy** and **counselling, autogenic training, naturopathy**, and **hyperthermia**. Results have shown some symptomatic improvements with possible reduction in both morbidity and mortality compared with patients treated with AZT. None of the patients having the AIDS-related complex (ARC) has yet progressed to full-blown AIDS.

Hay diet

A diet devised by American physician William Howard Hay (1866–1940) to treat digestive problems. He considered that protein stimulates the production of gastric acid, and since acid interferes with carbohydrate digestion it is preferable if carbohydrates are not eaten at the same time as acid foods such as fruits and protein. The principles of his diet are:

1 exclude peas, beans, lentils, and peanuts;

2 protein meals including meat, poultry, and fish and dairy products should be taken with acid fruits such as apples, oranges, apricots, and pears;

3 carbohydrate meals such as bread, flour, rice, and potatoes should be taken with non-acid fruits such as bananas, dates, and figs;

4 neutral foods such as nuts, vegetable oils, salads, and green and root vegetables can be combined with both protein and carbohydrate groups;

5 vegetables, salads, and fruits should form the major part of the diet, generally cutting down on proteins, starches, and fats;

6 no refined or processed foods should be included at all.

healing

A term which encompasses a wide range of techniques involving the beneficial influence of one person on another through mechanisms not recognized by orthodox medical science and without any form of mechanical or clinical manipulation. The 'laying on of hands' is usually regarded as a flow of energy from one person to another with the intention of curing illness, but may also involve the activation of the recipient's own self-healing abilities. Prayer and visualization by both the patient and the healer may help to focus positive thoughts on a patient's illness. Many healers make no attempt to diagnose a patient's illness, although in some cases the **aura** is examined or touch used to identify high and low energy areas. Controlled studies have shown beneficial effects from healing energies directed at bacteria, plants, cancer cells, and mice. There are many anecdotal reports of cures from untreatable illnesses, but in most cases healers do not function as an alternative to orthodox medical treatment.

healing mandala

A pattern of information wave-forms that automatically changes an environmental stress into a healing resonance. See also **mandala; resonance therapy**

health

A state in which all parts of the body are carrying out their proper functions and there is no malfunction present. There have been various attempts at definition:

World Health Organization (1947): Health is the complete state of physical, mental and social wellbeing, not merely the absence of disease.

Rene Dubois (1965): States of health are the expression of the success or failure experienced by the organism in its efforts to respond adaptively to environmental challenges.

Ivan Illich (1976): Health is the ability to adapt to changing environments — to growing up and to aging, to healing when damaged, to suffering, and to peaceful expectation of death.

health farm

A residential clinic which offers a wide variety of therapies, usually based on a naturopathic diet, which is mainly vegetarian and calorie-controlled, since many clients attend specifically to lose weight. Facilities generally include gymnasia, saunas, swimming pools, and outside recreations such as golf and tennis. Therapies include **acupuncture, aromatherapy, massage, reflexology, hydrotherapy**, and **osteopathy**.
See also **naturopathy**

health food

An imprecise term used to describe foods and dietary supplements which enjoy the reputation (deserved or otherwise) of being good for health. These foods are usually additive-free, but the term can be extended to include dietary supplements such as minerals, vitamins, trace elements, vegetable oils, and natural products such as evening primrose, castor oil, cod-liver oil and other fish oils, yoghurt, honey, royal jelly, and herbal remedies such as ginseng, gingko, angelica, and garlic. Many are sold simply as dietary supplements, but others may be claimed to have specific therapeutic effects.

healthwatch

An **electrical skin resistance** meter which is worn as a watch on the wrist and which measures skin resistance as an electric current is passed through it. This is used as a **biofeedback** instrument, and employs microchip technology developed by Walmsley Microsystems at Aston Science Park in Birmingham. High resistance indicates relaxation; low resistance indicates tension.

Healthwatch

An organization formerly called *Quackbusters*. It comprised a group of doctors and journalists who had the common aim of exposing malpractice, particularly fraud, in all forms of therapy including orthodox, alternative, and complementary medicine and of promoting the establishment of clinical trials to give an objective assessment of the effectiveness of various forms of therapy.

heather

A small evergreen shrub (*Calluna vulgaris*) found on moors and heathlands, the tiny flowers of which can be used to prepare a **Bach flower remedy** to help those people who are obsessed with, and never stop talking about, their own troubles.

Heller work

A form of deep tissue structural bodywork developed in 1978 by a former American aerospace engineer, Joseph Heller. His aim was to improve posture, movement, and breathing through a combination of manipulation, movement, and discussion with a view to releasing tension, relieving stress, and preventing illness.

herbal medicine

A herb is a plant that does not contain woody fibres (lignin), ie has no persistent parts above the ground. Herbalists use whole plants, or parts of plants, as remedies rather than separating out and concentrating the active ingredients. Plants have been eaten for their health-giving properties since prehistory. The Chinese pharmacopoeia dates from before 3000 BC, and Nicholas Culpeper (1616–54) wrote his

Herbal in 1653. Although many powerful drugs are now synthesized for use by orthodox medicine, approximately a third of all pharmaceutical products are still derived from plant sources. Herbal treatment is available for most kinds of illness, but is based on holistic assessment of the patient rather than just being prescribed symptomatically. Plant derivatives are highly active, and the active compounds may be concentrated in different parts of the plant. Seasons and the time of day may affect the best time for gathering. There are problems with standardizing herbal medicines, since they are complicated mixtures which may have hundreds of constituents rather than purified single agents. A computerized databank of published work is now available, and the British Herbal Medical Association Scientific Committee has produced a pharmacopoeia which is recognized by the government.
See also **phytotherapy**

HIV

The abbreviation for **H**uman **I**mmunodeficiency **V**irus, which is a *retrovirus* (so called because it enters the cell backwards). This is an RNA virus which copies its own genetic information into the DNA of the host, which then makes more viral RNA. It belongs to the subgroup *lentivirus*, which causes chronic slow virus diseases in animals (ie with a long incubation period). The virus enters the cell via a collection of special molecules on the surface membrane called GP120, which attaches to a cellular receptor (CD4) found mainly on the 'helper' lymphocytes. These lymphocytes are usually the first cells to respond to foreign antigen, since one of their functions is to switch on the other parts of the immune response. Their elimination can result in a breakdown of the immune system.
See also **AIDS; immune system**

holism

[Greek *holos* 'whole'] The view that a 'whole' cannot be defined fully in terms of its constituent parts. When applied to medicine, the holistic approach emphasizes that all aspects of a person are affected by an illness, and that effective treatment must be directed at the entire person and not just the diseased organ. Holistic treatment encourages a patient's capacity for self-healing, rather than resorting to surgical or drug treatment, and emphasizes education and self-care to achieve positive health rather than just the treatment of sickness. This involves proper diet, exercise, and lifestyle, and covers the entire range of mind, body, and spirit as well as social and other interactions. The term is derived from *Holism and Evolution* by Jan Christian Smuts (1926).

holly

A European evergreen tree or shrub (*Ilex aquifolia*) with white flowers and red berries from which a **Bach flower remedy** can be prepared. It is said to help to calm explosive feelings of envy, jealousy, hatred, revenge, and suspicion.

homeopathy

[Greek *homios* 'like'] A system of therapy based on the premise that substances which produce signs and symptoms in patients similar to those produced by a disease can also be used to cure them of that disease. The idea of treating 'like with like' was developed by German physician Samuel Hahnemann (1755–1843) in the early 1800s. He conducted clinical trials on remedies capable of producing artificial illnesses, which resulted in similar symptoms to those of the patient, thereby stimulating the patient's own defence mechanisms. The symptoms of disease represent the body's reaction to the illness, and should therefore be encouraged and not suppressed. The basic principles are that:

1 a medicine in large doses will produce symptoms like that of illness but in small doses will cure that illness;
2 by extreme dilution the undesirable effects of a medicine are lost, but its curative properties can be enhanced;
3 homeopathic medicines usually complement rather than substitute for orthodox medicines, and are prescribed individually from the study of the whole person (see **holism**) according to basic temperament, personality, reaction to the environment, and characteristics (*modalities*) of the illness.
See also **miasm**

homodot /hoʊmoʊˈdɒt/

A remedy produced from the liquid which results from the 'divide and recombining' process of **spagyrik therapy**. It is given to the patient in small amounts, thereby encouraging the body to correct its own dysfunction possibly by stimulating the immune response.

honeysuckle

A climbing shrub with tubular flowers which are often fragrant, especially at night, and from which a **Bach flower remedy** can be prepared. It is said to help those who are preoccupied with feelings of nostalgia and escapism, and who retreat into the past, being unable to focus on the present.

hornbeam

A deciduous tree (*Carpinus betulus*), common in coppices in the UK, with tiny flowers in the form of catkins from which a **Bach flower remedy** can be prepared. It is said to help those who procrastinate and who cannot face the thought of what lies ahead of them, responding with weariness and lethargy.

horseradish

Preparations from the plant *Armoracia rusticaria*, used for the treatment of toothache, neuralgia, coughs, and rheumatism. It is also said to prevent excessive lactation if applied to the breasts.

hospice

A type of hospital or nursing home specializing in the care of the terminally ill. The staff have particular expertise in dealing with all the personal needs of the patient, including emotional and spiritual problems and physical pain relief. The aim is to allow the patient to die without suffering and to help the relatives and loved ones to cope with the loss. In the Middle Ages hospices were hostels attached to monasteries which provided hospitality for travellers. The present-day hospice movement was started by a social worker who then trained to become a doctor, Dame Cicely Saunders (1918–   ), who founded St Christopher's Hospice in London in 1967 for patients with advanced or terminal cancer.

Hoxsey treatment /ˈhɒksi/

A cancer treatment developed by John Hoxsey in the 1840s based on a herbal tea, ointment, and powder which were made from the plants which a prize horse had chosen to eat when it was curing itself of a cancerous growth on its leg. He founded a clinic which also used herbs, vitamins, diet, interferon, immunotherapy, and live cell therapy against malignant disease.

humanistic psychotherapy

An approach to **psychotherapy** which emphasizes the importance of the person, rather than God's influence, or some other inanimate consideration; also known as *phenomenological psychotherapy*. It is concerned with the inner life of individuals, particularly with their current problems and their own feelings about themselves and the events surrounding them. The most important influences in this approach to psychology were Carl Rogers (1902–87) and Abraham Maslow (1908–70), who taught that each person is different and responsible for individual actions and behaviour. Patients are encouraged to explore concepts such as self-esteem, feelings, consciousness, and self-awareness.

hydrotherapy

The use of water for healing purposes by external or internal application. It is popular in continental Europe in health spas and hydros, particularly in Germany, Austria, and Switzerland. Water can be taken for medicinal purposes by mouth or by other routes, including colonic irrigation. External application may be by *bathing,* pressure hosing, the use of hot and cold towels, or underwater massage in which the body is submerged in a bath and massaged by strong jets of water. A hot bath can be used to produce an artificial fever as a way of removing toxic materials through the skin surface.
See also **hyperthermia; thalassotherapy**

hyperactivity

A syndrome seen in children, characterized by sleep disturbance, overactivity, lack of concentration, inattention, and poorly controlled behaviour. Dr Ben Feingold proposed early in the 1980s that hyperactivity was an ecological problem, in which additives and colourings in food were the cause of behavioural changes. It has also been seen in brain-damaged children and those with such disorders as autism and schizophrenia.

hyperthermia

A technique used in treating a wide variety of conditions, including cancer and AIDS, which is said to increase cell membrane permeability, increase the uptake of certain drugs, induce the death of heat sensitive cells, and enhance the body's immunological responses.

A high body temperature may be produced as a response to disease, infection, or deliberately induced to have beneficial effects. Artificial fever can be induced by the injection of foreign proteins or by radiant heat, diathermy, or hydro-therapy. Using a full immersion bath, temperature may be raised to 40–41°C, but the heart rate should be monitored and exposure not prolonged beyond 60 minutes. Children have poor temperature-regulating mechanisms, and patients with cardiovascular disease may also be at risk with hyperthermia treatment.
See also **hydrotherapy**

hypnoanalysis

The use of the state of **hypnosis** to allow the hypnotherapist to bypass the patient's conscious mind and communicate directly with the subconscious. This may be a useful way to encourage recollection of repressed memories and painful experiences.
See also **hypnosis**

hypnosis

An altered state of consciousness which is neither waking nor sleeping, usually induced by a therapist talking to a subject in a slow and controlled way and possibly requiring the subject to concentrate on an image. The result is a trance-like state of increased suggestibility and compliance. In deep hypnosis there is also a loss of pain sensation, which may be sufficient to allow surgical procedures to be carried out without other analgesia. In this altered state of mind patients may perform physical feats that they could not perform when conscious. It is possible to use hypnosis to access the subconscious mind and to implant post-hypnotic suggestions which may be activated by a predetermined signal after the patient has come out of the hypnotic state. Although this is an unreliable treatment technique, it has been used in the treatment of addiction to cigarettes, alcohol, and drugs, and for treating phobias, anxiety, and hysteria. The aims of the therapy are usually specified and agreed before the patient submits to hypnosis.

I

iatrogenic illness

[Greek *iatros* 'physician'+*genesis* 'origin'] An illness which arises as a direct result of medical treatment (for some other disease), such as the unwanted side effects of taking drugs. The treatments of **alternative medicine** are said to cause relatively fewer side effects than those of orthodox medicine, but there is little firm evidence to substantiate this belief.

immune system

A body defence system which detects and destroys harmful foreign substances (*allergens*), invading organisms (bacteria, fungi, viruses), and sometimes abnormal cells in the body (cancer cells, autoimmune disease). The specialized cells which perform this function constitute the *reticulo-endothelial system*, which includes the lymph nodes, spleen, and thymus gland. The result of their activity is to produce proteins called *antibodies* which can recognize and neutralize the antigens. Some cells (T cells, so called because they originate in the thymus gland) have the function of helping (T4) or suppressing (T8) antibody production or of killing harmful cells and pathogens directly (K cells or killer cells). The various components of this system communicate with each other by chemical transmitters including hormones and cytokines.
See also **AIDS; allergy; HIV**

immuno-augmentative therapy

A treatment giving *immune protein factors* which are extracted from the blood of volunteer donors (eg immunoglobulin concentrates) and sometimes from people who have suffered particular kinds of infection (eg hyperimmune globulin against measles, or cytomegalovirus). Some dramatic cancer cure claims have been made using plasma products derived from cancer sufferers.

immunosuppression

The suppression of the body's **immune system** using drugs such as cortico-steroids and cytotoxic agents, which kill dividing cells, and also radiation either to the whole body or just to the reticulo-endothelial system. This may be a deliberate strategy in treating auto-immune disorders or in achieving engraftment of transplanted tissue (eg kidney, heart, or bone marrow transplants). When people are immuno-suppressed, they are particularly susceptible to infections, and sometimes suffer severe or fatal infections from organisms which do not usually cause disease in healthy individuals (*opportunist infections*).

Impatiens

A genus of annual and perennial plants (including the 'Busy Lizzie') from which a **Bach flower remedy** can be prepared. It is said to calm those people who are always in a hurry and who show a tendency to impatience and irritability.

Indian medicine
See **ayurveda**

indigo

A red dye that comes from tropical shrubs (*indigofera*), said to stimulate intuition and imagination. It is associated with the 'third eye' and the brain's right hemisphere. Indigo persons are quiet, composed, and intuitive, but sometimes have unrealistic ideas about themselves. They often join the healing professions.
See also **colour therapy**

infusion

A drink prepared by adding boiling water to fresh or dried herbs, either loose or in bags, and allowing the mixture sufficient time for the soluble constituents to enter solution (usually 10–15 minutes) before drinking.

inhalation therapy

The inhalation of steam (from boiling water), often with aromatic oils such as eucalyptus or menthol added to the water. Steam inhalation is recommended for unblocking sinuses and clearing catarrh. Orthodox medicine may recommend the use of an 'inhaler', which releases a limited dose of a drug in aerosol suspension or fine powder form as the patient takes a deep breath. Such devices are particularly used for treating asthma and other chest conditions, but only 10–15% of the inhaled drug actually ends up in the lungs, most of it being deposited on the back of the throat.

integral psychoanalysis

A system of psychoanalysis founded by Norberto R Keppe in Brazil in 1970, based on his philosophy that human consciousness is a synthesis of feelings (love), thought (truth), and 'real action' (correct action), directed by goodness, beauty, and truth. The process of recognizing harmful attitudes and deliberately correcting them include *conscientization* of error. He proposed that human suffering is the result of individual and social attitudes interfering with a person's freedom to take 'real action'.

intellectual rhythm

A biorhythm affecting perception, learning, and powers of reasoning and argument. In a positive phase one can think constructively and take correct decisions, but in a negative phase errors of judgement may be made.
See also **biorhythms**

intolerance

An adverse reaction of the body to an external stimulus which is not usually noxious to other people (eg food or drug intolerance). Sometimes there are psychological factors which may result in or aggravate intolerance.

ionizer

An electrical apparatus that generates negative charges which are taken up by airborne particles (eg smoke and dust), and which are then attracted to the ground, walls, and other (positively charged) surfaces, thus clearing the air. Most air particles are electrically neutral, but negative ions are generated by running water, ocean waves, lightning, and the effects of radiation from the sun and outer space. Pollution and the electrical activity from electrical appliances, central heating, and air conditioners all destroy negative charges. Ionizers may be helpful for people suffering from respiratory problems, skin allergies, headaches, hay fever, catarrh, depression, and insomnia. Some manufacturers also claim improvements in alertness and concentration, together with a feeling of well-being.

See also **air imbalance; electro-pollution; negative ion therapy**

iridology

The detailed study of the visible parts of the eye, especially the iris; also called *ophthalmic somatology*. Iridologists claim that the whole body is reflected in the appearance of the eyes, since the nervous system comes to the surface at this point. Detailed examination can thus reveal physical and psychological problems as well as evidence of past disorders and tendencies towards future illness. In 1950 American physician Bernard Jensen constructed a map of the iris showing its correlation with the rest of the body, which may be used as a diagnostic aid in conjunction with many therapies including acupuncture, herbal medicine, and homeopathy. The colour of the eyes is genetically determined, and can show a predisposition to particular illnesses. A blue iris is called *lymphatic*, and these people have a tendency to respiratory problems and rheumatism. A brown iris is called *haematogenic*, and reveals a tendency to blood and circulatory problems.

iron balls

Chinese hollow iron balls, available in a range of sizes but which are small enough to be rotated in the palms of the hands. They provide exercise for the fingers and wrists.

Usually two balls are used, which may be engraved and ornamented, or contain chimes sounding high (**yin**) and low (**yang**). The action of the balls in the palm of the hand stimulates acupuncture points connected with the heart and other major organs, and in this way the exercises improve circulation and calm the mind and body.

J

jade

A semi-precious stone in many shades of green which may be either *jadeite*, a single chain silicate structure which is relatively rare, or *nephrite*, a complex hydrous double-chained silicate with a waxy lustre. It is greatly prized in China, where it was used for ornamental carving and jewellery, and is also found in the New World, particularly in Mexico. It is a soft gentle stone which brings good luck and is said to promote friendship, flexibility, tolerance, and a long, prosperous life.
See also **crystal therapy**

jin shin do /ˈdʒɪn ʃɪn ˈdoʊ/

A form of **acupressure** which concentrates on the 'eight extra meridians', rather than using points on the classical acupuncture channels. These extra meridians are said to act as a reservoir of energy, and to contain the vital essence which is derived from the kidneys. For this reason, their use is thought to allow a deeper level of treatment, which can act on a patient's basic constitution, and affect energy at its deepest levels.

jogging

A popular form of exercise which involves running at a pace defined as being slow enough to allow a conversation. Although generally safe in terms of serious health risks, sprains and muscle strain may occur, and haemoglobinuria can result from repeated trauma to the soles of the feet if protective shoes and socks are not worn.

K

karma

[Sanskrit, 'action, work'] In the Indian tradition, the name given to the law of cause and effect (ie there is a reaction to every action). The results of our actions are believed to be carried forward from one life to the next, with consequent improvement or deterioration in our fate. The purpose of life is to learn through successive incarnations to develop our potential to the full, and to fulfil our spiritual destiny. A knowledge of previous incarnations can help to plan the present life and to avoid repeating the mistakes that have been made before. This is the purpose of karmic astrology.

Kilner screen

A screen made from two pieces of glass which enclose an indigo-violet coloured fluid (*dicyanin*). This absorbs part of the visual spectrum and allows a practitioner of **colour therapy** to see a patient's **aura** more clearly. Ideally the patient should wear a black silk robe so as not to distract the practitioner's vision.

kinesics /kaɪˈniːzɪks/

[Greek *kinesis* 'motion'] The study of body language as a method of communication, including the use of facial expressions, gestures, movements, and postures. There may be marked discrepancies in the use made of certain gestures among different cultures.

kinesiology

[Greek *kinesis* 'motion'] A system of diagnosis and treatment developed by American chiropractor George Goodheart, based on the idea that each group of muscles is related to other distant parts of the body and that a patient's muscular response to manual pressure allows the practitioner to detect blockages and imbalances and to localize physical problems.

Diagnosis is often based on **traditional Chinese medicine**, and balance is achieved using the classical 12 **acupuncture meridians** which are identical with the *kinesiology channels* by applying finger tip massage to 'pressure points' to enhance blood, lymphatic, and energy (**qi**) flow to the muscles. A well-known application is for allergy testing, when food, chemicals, or other possible **allergens** are placed in the hand and on the tongue, and this is said to affect muscle power and the body's electrical field.

See also **systematic kinesiology; touch for health**

Kirlian photography

A technique which uses a very high voltage (30000–50000 volts), but with negligible current flowing, to create a high intensity electric field that allows electrons to break away from surfaces. These electrons can then be recorded on a photographic plate as a record of the electrical interference pattern. Materials which are good conductors will show only the surface of the object, but poor conductors show detail of their inner structure. Dead objects have a constant outline, whereas living objects show a constantly changing pattern which is said to reveal the physical and psychological state of the subject. The phenomenon was discovered by Russian engineer Semeyon Kirlian and his wife Valentina in 1939 (published in 1961), and in 1991 Dr Philippe Dien of Belgium developed a diagnostic system in which Kirlian photographs of the feet and hands, together with a clinical history and blood samples, are referred to a central laboratory in Paris for diagnosis and treatment formulation. These results may be used as a counselling tool to assess a person's energy balance, to monitor what is happening to their 'subtle energy' fields, and to assess possible responses to treatment. Cancer tissue, for example, is said to show a characteristic *coronal discharge*. There has up to now been a lack of objective assessment of these energies, and attention is currently focusing on computer enhancement and evaluation of these patterns.

See also **bioelectrography**

koan /ˈkoʊɑːn/

A paradox or parable which cannot be explained using the logical mind. It is used as an aid to meditation to free students

from the confines of a rational mind by confronting them with a problem which can only be responded to by insight and not with reason. An example is: 'What is the sound of one hand clapping?'
See also **Zen**

ko cycle
The controlling or interacting cycle in which each element controls or is controlled by another element, resulting in a self-regulating balance:

wood controls earth, ie liver controls spleen;
earth controls water, ie spleen controls kidney;
water controls fire, ie kidney controls heart;
fire controls metal, ie heart controls lung;
metal controls wood, ie lung controls liver.
See also **five elements**

kundalini /kʊndə'liːni/
[Sanskrit, 'serpentine, twisting force'] The sexual energy which rises up the centre channel of the spine to the brain, where it awakens spiritual illumination and inner perception.

kunzite
An orchid pink gemstone, discovered in 1902. It is said to rejuvenate the tissues and activate the heart. It is also a feminine stone which encourages self-love and acceptance and may help regulate menstrual problems.

kuzu
A vegetable powder used to thicken sauces, soups and desserts, which is said to help settle the digestive system.
See also **macrobiotics**

L

Laetrile /ˈlaɪtrɪl/

A trade name for the drug *amygdalin* (bitter almond), found in some fruit stones, such as apricot. It is regarded as dangerous, as it produces cyanide in the body. Formerly called vitamin $B_1 7$, it was promoted as a cancer cure in 1970 by pathologist Ernesto Contreras in Tijuana, Mexico as part of his metabolic therapy. Laetrile may be recommended to prevent cancer in high-risk situations such as people who have a family history, or who are exposed to a hazardous occupation or environment, but it is not regarded as effective by orthodox medicine. See also **Manner therapy**

lapis lazuli

A deep blue stone, once the source of the pigment ultramarine, containing a mixture of sodium and aluminium silicate. Regarded as the royal stone in Ancient Egypt, and the stone of the gods, it is said to open the mind to divine wisdom and inner vision, and to represent truth and integrity. See also **crystal therapy**

larch

A deciduous conifer found in the northern hemisphere from which a **Bach flower remedy** can be prepared. It is said to help those who lack self-confidence and consequently miss opportunities, even though they have the capability to take them up.

laser therapy

Laser is an abbreviation of *light amplification by stimulated emission of radiation*. The laser beam is a high-energy electromagnetic wave generated in either solid (ruby) liquid (dyes in solvents) or gaseous (helium/neon, argon/krypton) phases. The light is composed of photons identical in phase and moving in the same direction, so that it is monochromatic and does not spread out, thus producing a high-intensity beam which is undiminished over large distances.

Laser beams have been used in scanning, welding, hologram production, weapon systems, medicine, and surgery. They may also be used to stimulate acupuncture points, and this allows treatment of patients who would not normally tolerate needles (especially children). The commonest machine for this purpose is a helium-neon laser (*theralaser*) which produces an infra-red beam via a hand-held 'pencil' with a power of 2 milliwatts. It may be used either for irradiating specific points for 60–90 seconds or with stroking and waving movements along meridians.

laughter

A complicated action which combines a facial expression comprising the baring of teeth and screwing up of the face with increased rhythmic breathing and the making of inarticulate sounds. It is taken as a sign of friendliness, welcoming, and humour, stimulates the circulation, and increases the level of arousal hormones including adrenaline and noradrenalin. The initial stimulation of laughter is followed by a period of relaxation and loss of tension, and it provides important mental, emotional, spiritual, and physical benefits. Because of its beneficial effects, attempts have been made to use laughter as a therapeutic technique.

lavender

A plant (*Lavendula officinalis*) which belongs to the mint family, whose leaves can be processed to yield an essential oil. The name is derived from Latin (*lavare* 'to wash'), and lavender water baths were popular with the Romans. Posies of lavender were used to protect against bad air and noxious smells in 19th-century London. Lavender is the basis for the preparation of eau de cologne, and the essential oil is said to have a harmonizing effect which is useful in treating all kinds of stress. The action of the oil depends upon the needs of the recipient, and can be both stimulant and warming or sedative and cooling. Other reported uses include accelerating wound healing, stimulating the immune system, and acting as an antiseptic.

laying on of hands

The action of placing the hands on or near a sick person, with the intention of curing their mental or physical illness. The early Christians developed this technique following the example of Jesus Christ as a way of channelling the power of God or the Holy Spirit to cure the sick.

Le Boyer method

A method of natural childbirth developed by American physician Frederick Le Boyer (1918–   ). It emphasizes that a baby should enter the world as gently as possible and that the delivery should be conducted with subdued lighting and quiet so that the infant does not experience unpleasant sensations at birth.

Lesh states

A classification of the levels of relaxation attained during meditation, as described by American physician Terry Lesh at the University of Oregon:

State 0 difficulty in stilling the mind, and distracted by everyday thoughts;
State 1 drifting into a daydream, and forgetting the objective of relaxing or meditating;
State 2 calmness but not able to sustain attention;
State 3 sustained concentration with a body sensation of floating, swaying, or lightness;
State 4 an enhanced awareness of body sensations such as breathing and heartbeat;
State 5 intense alertness, calmness, and detachment;
State 6 a new way of feeling.

lettuce

An annual or perennial plant (*Lactuca sativa*) widely used in salads. Eating fresh lettuce or drinking the water in which lettuce has been boiled are both said to relieve insomnia.

ley lines

[From an Anglo-Saxon word meaning 'a cleared strip of land']
A term applied in 1921 by Alfred Watkins to lines connecting
ancient sites and features across the countryside (eg burial
mounds, standing stones). These lines were originally
thought to be ancient trading tracks, but have recently been
described as 'energy lines' which can be detected and mapped
by **dowsing**. Another theory is that they represent 'spirit lines'
or ghost paths which begin and end in cemeteries.

light therapy

A therapeutic technique which makes use of artificial light.
The average intensity of daylight is 5000 lux, but indoor light
is only 500 lux. The minimum intensity required to influence
the body's hormones and neurochemical mechanisms is 2500
lux. Adequate light is essential for the production of vitamin
D and to stimulate the immune system. A *light box* may be
used to simulate daylight, and emits approximately 2500 lux.
Light boxes have been used successfully to treat **seasonal
affective disorder (SAD)** and premenstrual tension. Light
therapy is also helpful for night-shift workers and for those
suffering depression, fatigue, and sleeping difficulty. It is a
non-invasive therapy with no adverse side effects.

liquorice

A perennial plant (*Glycyrrhiza glabra*) cultivated for its roots
which are used both in confectionery and medicine. The root
and stem may be chewed raw, reduced by crushing, or boiled
and then the juice evaporated to prepare liquid, powder, and
lozenges. Liquorice acts as a soothing agent, an anti-
spasmodic to relieve stomach pains, and a laxative. It also has
anti-inflammatory, antibacterial, and anti-allergic properties, and can act as an expectorant by increasing the
production of sputum and by its mucolytic action.

live cell therapy

A treatment, developed in the 1970s in a Swiss clinic, which is
claimed to stimulate the regeneration of damaged or diseased
tissues and cells. Freshly prepared foetal tissue of unborn
calves, lambs, and pigs, which corresponds to the diseased

organs being treated (eg cartilage and synovial membrane for joint disease), are administered by intramuscular injection. There are some anecdotal accounts of beneficial effects, but no proper studies have been conducted. The injection of foreign protein is potentially hazardous, and there may also be a danger of virus transmission. The treatment is also known as *cellular therapy*.

lucerne
See **alfalfa**

luminaissance
A form of holistic midwifery developed by Anne and Michel Bercot in Paris in the mid-1980s 'to welcome newly incarnating souls into life'. They emphasize the spiritual nature of the child, and avoid damaging factors such as over-medication during the birth process and medically-created trauma in childhood. They aim to educate the parents to recognize and care for the child's spiritual nature.

Luscher colour test
A personality test devised by Dr Max Luscher based on colour preferences and the premise that preferred colours reflect the personality. The test consists of scoring colours in order of preference.

lymphatic drainage
A method of massage which is said to encourage the flow of lymph and activate the lymphatic system by massaging along lymphatic channels. It is also said to stimulate the para-sympathetic nervous system, which may improve rest and sleep and relieve stress. Beneficial effects have also been reported in relieving the symptoms of oedema and some skin problems.

M

macrobiotics

A philosophy of life originated by Sagen Ishizuka in the 1880s, following **Zen** Buddhist principles, which takes a wide (*macro*) view of life (*biotic*) and emphasizes the benefits of wholesome behaviour and eating. A set of dietary principles ('a perfect diet') was formulated based on the careful balance of **yin** and **yang** to select the ideal foods necessary for long-term health. The diet is based on vegetables and whole-grain cereals, including brown rice. No processed food is allowed, and very little meat is used. Where possible, foodstuffs are kept alive until cooked, and their individual character is maintained by delaying the mixing of foods until the last moment before serving. The system was popularized by the Japanese writer George Ohsawa, who claimed that this dietary system had cured his TB. He then embarked upon a world-wide tour promoting the macrobiotic approach. Some critics say that such a diet lacks protein, and so is inappropriate for children.

magma

A health-food supplement particularly recommended for use when convalescing from a long illness. It consists of a mixture of brown rice with freshly cut and spray-dried barley leaves from organically grown plants.

magnetic therapy

A therapeutic technique using magnetic fields. Paracelsus, in the 16th century, said that 'the magnet is very useful in treating internal and external diseases'. More recently magnetic fields have been shown to affect cell permeability, enabling nutrients to enter the cells and toxins to leave. Pulsating magnetic fields induce low frequency currents in the tissues, and work at the Institute of Medical Science in Munich has shown a beneficial effect on the healing of fractures. Less substantiated claims have been made for accelerated wound healing with reduction in scar tissue, and for improvement in blood circulation to the extremities with lowering of blood pressure. Personal Magnetic Therapy devices can now be purchased, and are advertised for the relief of rheumatism, arthritis, migraine, muscular tension, and respiratory and gynaecological problems. These machines can be used safely for 24 hours a day if required, but stronger permanent magnets and the use of pulsed electro-magnetic energy (PEME) require the expertise of trained therapists and equipment not suited to home use. Magnets are sometimes applied to reflexology or acupuncture points, but so far reports on the efficacy of these treatments are entirely anecdotal.

See also **biomagnetics**

malachite
A brilliant green stone (hydrated copper carbonate) which is said to balance the physical body, and is used as a talisman against falling over. It strengthens and protects the heart chakra, and clears the mind of illusions. It is said to be good for rheumatism and arthritis, and to have antiseptic and anti-inflammatory effects.

See also **crystal therapy**

mandala
A pattern or design, usually taken from Buddhist or Hindu art, which often represents the universe. It is used as an aid to meditation.

manipulation
[Latin *manipulare* 'to handle', ie treatment by hand] A set of techniques usually practised by physiotherapists, chiropractors, and osteopaths to improve the mobility of joints and soft tissues, decrease muscle spasm, and relieve pain. Sometimes the term is restricted to high velocity thrusts applied to joints, and these techniques may be carried out under anaesthetic to ensure complete relaxation if excessive pain is anticipated or if fibrosis has previously limited the range of movements. Manipulation is generally contra-indicated in malignant and inflammatory diseases of bones and soft tissues.

See also **chiropractic; osteopathy**

manipura

The third **chakra**, situated behind the umbilicus and linked with the solar plexus, and also with the stomach, spleen, liver, gall bladder, and muscles. The 'vital essence' is consumed at this centre, which leads to old age and decay. Its actions are connected with the eyes and sight, and with the feet and physical activity. If the manipura chakra is unstable, there may be mood swings with depression and introversion, and an abnormal appetite but with poor digestion.

Manner therapy

A type of therapy developed by American physician Harold Manner, who is now Head of the Metabolic Research Foundation. The therapy, *metabolic cancer therapy*, is based on a diet with supplements which include vitamins A and C and digestive enzymes, together with the use of **Laetrile**.

mantra

[Sanskrit *man+tra* 'instrument of thought'] A sacred word, or group of words, especially from the Vedas, originally used in prayers and incantations. More recently the repetition of mantras has been used as an aid to meditation, and is reputed to help the development of spiritual powers.

marmalade

[Portuguese *marmeto* 'quince'] A type of fruit preserve made by boiling the fruit with sugar. A popular story associated with the name derives it from the French *Marie est malade*, referring to a dish of sweet boiled quinces which was prepared for Mary, Queen of Scots when she was sick. Nowadays marmalade is usually made from Seville **oranges**, and is popular in Britain as a breakfast preserve taken on toast.

masked sensitivity

A condition in which an allergy to a foodstuff (or other allergy) is present but not obvious, and becomes apparent only after a period of fasting. The sensitivity can be demonstrated by an **elimination diet** in which a patient fasts for five days, and then foods are reintroduced one by one. Under these circumstances (the 'hyperacute state') there may be severe reactions within a few minutes of ingesting a food allergen.
See also **allergy**

massage

A series of techniques for soft tissue manipulation, performed with the subject relaxed and passive, to relax and tonify the muscles. Massage is often used in conjunction with other therapies such as aromatherapy, acupuncture, reflexology, and orthodox medical treatment, and can promote good health by stimulating and invigorating both mind and body. See also **Thai massage**

McTimoney chiropractic

A gentle form of whole body manipulation to correct misalignments in the spinal column and other joints, and which may alleviate pain, restore nerve function, and promote good health.

ME

See **myalgic encephalomyelitis**

meditation

[Sanskrit *medha* 'wisdom'] A variety of techniques which attempt to control thought processes and calm the body by using powers of concentration. This may be undertaken purely for relaxation and to calm the mind, or as a way of achieving spiritual enlightenment either within or outside the framework of religion. Factors common to all techniques involve a deep relaxation of all muscle groups, awareness of breathing, and a passive attitude which is associated with reduced activity in the sympathetic nervous system and a tranquil state of mind and body. Some techniques employ the repetition of selected sounds (a **mantra**) synchronized with the breathing.

megavitamin therapy

A logical extension of corrective diet therapies which assumes that some patients (eg cancer patients) may not be able to absorb adequate quantities of vitamins and minerals from their diets, and require much larger amounts than usual. American chemist and Nobel Prize winner Linus Pauling (1901–) advocated large doses of vitamin C to prevent or cure the common cold, postulating both immune enhancement and a direct antiviral effect when used in large doses. Megavitamin therapy has been particularly applied in psychiatry, on the assumption that some mental disorders may be due to vitamin deficiencies, and case reports of beneficial effects in patients with schizophrenia, depression, and hyperactivity in children have been published. Some vitamins may cause toxic effects when given in excessive amounts.

See also **orthomolecular medicine**

meridians

Channels or pathways through which **qi** energy flows and along the courses of which **acupuncture** points are located. There are 12 principal meridians, linked to the internal organs, which are paired (right and left sides) and named after the organs with which they are associated. There are also 8 'extra' meridians which are not directly linked to organs; these do not have acupuncture points in their own right, but are routed between points on the principal meridians.

mesmerism

A technique named after Austrian physician Franz Anton Mesmer (1734–1815) who held public demonstrations of hypnosis in France during the 1780s. He believed that all illness was caused by imbalances in animal magnetism, which he defined as the energy involved in the hypnotic state. Many subjects reported improvements following his demonstrations; these people were most likely to have been suffering from psychosomatic illnesses amenable to cure by suggestion.

metamorphic technique

A holistic method of treatment developed in the 1960s by British naturopath Robert St John (1912–   ) based upon **reflexology**. He believes that the reflex areas related to the spine reflect pre-natal development, which in turn affects the

subject's physical and psychological characteristics. When the practitioner touches reflex points on the feet, hands, and head, the patient's own energies are encouraged to rebalance themselves.
See also **naturopathy**

miasm /'maɪəzm/

[Greek *miainein* 'to pollute'] A persistent distortion of the body's energy fields which may lead to disease or increased susceptibility to seemingly unrelated conditions. The concept was developed by the founder of homeopathy, Samuel Hahnemann (1755–1843).

Miasms may be inherited, possibly as the result of an infectious illness suffered by an ancestor which may influence their genetic function and hence cause maldevelopment in subsequent generations. Acquired miasms usually result from acute infectious illness in which, although the acute phase passes, a toxic influence may persist to give rise to chronic symptoms.

Inherited and acquired miasms are of great importance in **psionic medicine** but the energy distortions described are detectable only by 'supersensible' methods.
See also **homeopathy**

mimulus

A ubiquitous annual or perennial plant having yellow flowers with splashes of red, from which a **Bach flower remedy** can be prepared. It is recommended for those people who are usually shy, nervous, and retiring, and who fear various aspects of everyday life.

mineral therapy

A therapeutic technique based on the use of mineral supplements in the diet. A well-balanced diet should provide all the necessary essential nutrients, including minerals; in some circumstances (eg poor diet, malabsorption, pregnancy, or blood loss) deficiencies may develop which can cause illness. Dietary advice and mineral supplements may be required, and many compound preparations are now widely available containing essential trace elements. However, excessive consumption of trace elements may also lead to illness.

The term *mineral therapy* is also used to describe a system of treatment developed by Dr William Schuessler in 1873, who taught that normal cell metabolism, which is necessary for health, depends upon a supply of nutrients including essential 'mineral tissue salts'. He described 12 vital mineral tissue salts, and prescribed homeopathic doses of these minerals, usually at a six-times dilution to restore normal function.
See also **homeopathy**

miso /ˈmiːzəʊ/
A seasoning, like soy sauce, made from fermented soya beans. It is said to strengthen the blood and aid digestion.

mistletoe
An evergreen shrub (*Viscum album* of the family *Loranthaceae*) which grows as a parasite usually upon deciduous trees. Mistletoe was regarded as a sacred plant by the Druids, who cut it from oak trees with a golden knife and regarded it as a panacea, with particular activity against infertility and as an antidote to poisons. More recently an extract of mistletoe has been shown to have a cytotoxic effect which may be useful in treating cancer, and this work forms the basis of the 'Iscador' treatment practised by Swiss homeopath and naturopath, Alfred Vogel.

mobilization
A form of manipulation which includes traction or stretching along the longitudinal axis of a tissue and rotation through the available range of movement of a joint. Repetitive passive movements are designed to relax muscles, relieve pain, and stretch tight tissues.

modalities
The detailed characteristics of a patient and their an illness which define or 'qualify' a symptom. They allow a homeopathic physician to select the most appropriate remedy.
See also **homeopathy**

Moerman therapy

A treatment for cancer following the principles of Dutch physician Cornelius Moerman. He believes that dietary management, especially of vitamin and mineral supplements which aim to increase the body's oxidation capacity, will help to destroy tumours.

See also **mineral therapy**

monilia

See **candida**

moonstone

A white, opalescent, semi-precious gemstone form of feldspar, associated with the goddess Diana. It is said to be good for the pituitary gland and for developing emotional sensitivity. It arouses passion and opens the heart when exchanged between lovers.

See also **crystal therapy**

moxa

A term derived from the Japanese name for the plant *Artemesia vulgaris*, which belongs to the chrysanthemum family. The dried leaves are used in the form of moxa sticks (rolled leaves), moxa cones, and 'punk', a dry fibrous substance with a wool-like consistency which can be rolled and applied to **acupuncture** needles.

See also **moxibustion**

moxibustion

A technique for applying local heat over **acupuncture** points either indirectly by heating needles, or directly using **moxa** cones (placed on the skin over the points) or moxa sticks (held over the points at a distance from the skin surface). The technique originated in the cold mountainous regions of northern China, and probably preceded the use of needles. Heat penetrates deeply, affecting the flow of **qi** and supplementing it. It is particularly beneficial for cold and chronic painful conditions such as arthritis.

mud therapy

A therapeutic technique using certain types of mud, which contain beneficial substances of mineral and plant origin. When applied to the surface of the skin, these substances may penetrate the skin and enter the blood stream. The application of mud, in the form of mud packs, encourages sweating, rids the body of impurities, and invigorates the skin by abrasion. It is said to be particularly useful for rheumatism, arthritis, and gynaecological problems.

muesli

A popular high-fibre, low-fat, breakfast cereal, available in a wide variety of mixtures of cereals, nuts, and fruits. Dr Max Bircher-Benner (1867–1939) ran a clinic in Zürich where he used a raw food diet which was the forerunner of modern muesli, and included a mixture of oatmeal, grated apples, berries, and milk.

muladhara /mʊˈlædrə/

The root or base **chakra**, situated at the tip of the coccyx in the peritoneum. It is closely linked with the urogenital system, particularly the prostate gland and testicles in the male and uterus in the female. This chakra is the seat of the **kundalini** or sexual energy.

music

Music is used as a form of psychotherapy for relaxation, helping to cope with stress and providing a route to deeper feelings. It may help with breath control and can be used in conjunction with various forms of exercise and as an aid to meditation. Music may have profound effects on the emotions of the listener, and can be a powerful means of self-expression for those performing.

mustard

An annual plant (*Brassica alba*) with yellow flowers from which a **Bach flower remedy** can be prepared. This is said to help those who are suffering from depression which descends upon them like a cloud, bringing sadness and misery without any apparent reason.

myalgic encephalomyelitis (ME)

A syndrome whose most common clinical components are extreme exhaustion, muscle pains aggravated by exercise, stomach upset, and psychological features which are made worse by stress, including difficulty in concentrating, mood swings, and depression; also known as *chronic fatigue syndrome, post-viral fatigue syndrome,* and *chronic fatigue immunodeficiency syndrome.* Some consistent features under investigation include persistent enterovirus infection (eg with ECHO and Coxsackie B), and depressed immunological responses. The condition often starts as a flu-like illness from which complete recovery does not occur. It has been suggested that a period of stress on or around the time of a viral infection may impair the immune response and prevent complete recovery.

myrobalan

See **cherry plum**

N

naprapathy

[Czech *napra* 'fix'+Greek *pathos* 'suffering'] A form of bodywork developed by American osteopath Oakley Smith in Chicago at the turn of the century. The basic principle is that trauma can cause a blockage which interferes with the blood and nerve supply to an area, with misalignment of the connective tissue around joints. Examination concentrates on palpating all around the joints of the body for tension, pain, and restriction of movement. Treatment consists of stretching the muscles and connective tissues to allow correction of bony misalignments. This form of connective tissue bodywork may also improve the function of related internal organs.

narcoanalysis

The use of small doses of anaesthetic drugs to render a patient drowsy yet still able to communicate. In this state inhibitions may be removed which can allow the therapist to explore emotional problems which would not usually be accessible. This technique may be used in conjunction with various forms of **psychotherapy**.

natural childbirth

The delivery of children without artificial aids, ie with minimal use of drugs and assistance. The technique was pioneered by British physician Grantly Dick-Reed (1890–1959). It is said to be less traumatic for the baby, and to give women more control over the birth process. There is no particular favoured position for childbirth, and delivery may be conducted in squatting, sitting, or even standing up positions, since lying down causes mechanical difficulties. The National Childbirth Trust provides counselling and classes about posture, exercise, and diet to assist women in their preparation for natural childbirth both physically and psychologically.

natural reconnective therapy

A form of gentle soft tissue manipulation, to eliminate the stresses accumulated in connective tissues, brought to the UK from France in 1986 by Annick Labouré and Pierre Marion. The method includes nutritional and lifestyle modifications, including getting to bed early five nights per week and taking only two meals per day, with the main meal before 9.00 am and a smaller one at noon.

naturopathy

An approach to health care and treatment characterized by the following principles:

1 the body possesses the power to heal itself; treatment is not a question of eliminating an illness but rather of inducing the presence of health;
2 the symptoms of disease are a manifestation of the healing process, the result of the body's attempt to correct its disturbed equilibrium; it is therefore inappropriate to suppress symptoms;
3 a holistic approach to health care and treatment is required, which may involve a complete reorganization of the patient's lifestyle. Treatment usually begins with fasting to eliminate toxins, and proceeds to a natural diet which includes whole and unrefined foods with fruit and juices to consolidate the benefits of the fasting and maintain good health. This is combined with systematic exercise and education about the basic principles of nutrition, hygiene, and lifestyle, to encourage patients to take responsibility for their own illnesses.

needling sensation

The sensation induced by the insertion of an **acupuncture** needle when the acupuncture point is accurately located and the **qi** is stimulated. This sensation is not usually painful, but may be described as dull, heavy, or tingling and may possibly radiate up or down the related meridian. Traditionalists believe that inducing this sensation is essential to achieve the maximum therapeutic effects from acupuncture.
See also **meridians**

negative ion therapy

The use of negatively-charged air particles to prevent and cure disease. Country and mountain air contains a high concentration of negative ions (>1000 per ml). The air in cities has a lower ion concentration (100–500 per ml), and inside air-conditioned buildings there may be a predominance of positive ions which can cause restlessness, anxiety, depression, headaches, and irritability. Negative ion generators use high voltage discharges, ultra-violet light and water sprays. NASA use negative ionizers in the atmosphere of their spacecraft to improve the performance and work capacity of their crews. Some well-documented effects of negatively-ionized air include a reduction in heart rate and blood pressure, increased tidal volume of air breathed, and increased muco-ciliary action. Negative ions affect circulating hormone levels and brain-wave patterns, and have been used to treat psychoneurosis as well as headaches, asthma, bronchitis, and skin problems. Ions may be applied by breathing ionized air or by directing ions on to an affected area.

See also **ionizer**

Nei Ching

An abbreviation of *Huang Ti Nei Ching*, the Yellow Emperor's Classic of Internal Medicine, a book compiled from c.500 BC and eventually recorded in approximately AD 100. It lists the principles and therapies of **traditional Chinese medicine**, beginning in the reign of the Yellow Emperor (approximately 2700 BC), and includes an account of the organ functions of the **zang fu** and their interrelationship, the theory of **yin** and **yang**, the **five elements** (or five phases), diet, diagnosis, breathing exercises, and **acupuncture**.

neurolinguistic programming (NLP)

A system which aims to improve the ability to communicate, to achieve rapid learning, and to encourage behaviour changes in oneself and others. The system's name comes from neurolinguistics, the study of the way in which the brain controls speech and comprehension, and was developed from the work of psychotherapists Milton Erickson, Fritz Perls, and Virginia Satir, based on their studies of how outstanding individuals manage to achieve their states of excellence. They developed a theory to explain how the brain organizes and stores information, and how this can be used to improve behaviour patterns and change destructive habits. The training methods aim to develop inner strengths and abilities, and to resolve past hurts and conflicts, and may be integrated with other therapeutic approaches.

nine remedies

The nine methods used to adjust the circulation of **qi** both inside and outside a building to harmonize with the environment.

1 bright objects, eg mirrors, crystal balls;
2 sound, eg wind chimes;
3 living objects, eg plants, fish in tanks;
4 moving objects, eg water fountains;
5 heavy objects, eg statues and stones;
6 flutes;
7 electrical power;
8 colours;
9 a view of water.

nosode complexes /ˈnɒzoʊd/

Homeopathic remedies which are prepared from the discharges produced during illnesses caused by bacteria, viruses, chemicals, and allergens. Nosodes may be either single, from a specific organism or toxin, or complexes containing a mixture of substances. Nosode complexes are used to treat the after-effects of the related illness.
See also **homeopathy**

numerology

The study of the symbolic qualities of numbers, mainly derived from Hindu and Arabic teaching, but also found in the Jewish and Chinese traditions. In the Chinese tradition odd numbers are **yang** and represent the celestial world, bringing good fortune, whereas even numbers are **yin**, representing receptivity and the terrestrial world. The European belief is based mostly on the works of Pythagoras, who felt that the character of each of the nine numbers (like the letters of the alphabet) is linked to cosmic influences, and that numerology can be used to assess the energies available at a particular time, ie the hour, day, week, month, and year.

nutritional medicine

The study of the way nutrients nourish the body, including the physiology of their digestion, absorption, and utilization by the body. The practice of traditional medicine is based upon an orthodox medical assessment with history, physical examination, and possibly further laboratory tests to establish a diagnosis, eg the measurement of vitamin and mineral levels, or the assessment of bowel function using absorption tests. Treatment is given by avoiding any identified allergens, desensitization against offending food items, and the correction of any deficiencies demonstrated using appropriate supplements. The clinical application of knowledge of the interactions between nutritional factors and human metabolism can be used to improve health and strengthen the constitution to prevent and treat disease. This is particularly important for preconceptual and prenatal care.

O

oak

A large deciduous tree (genus *Quercus*) from whose flowers a **Bach flower remedy** can be prepared. It is said to help those who are strong, courageous, and reliable, but who have lost their strength through illness or adversity and are consequently annoyed with themselves.

oleander

A highly poisonous evergreen shrub (*Nerium oleander*) with purple, pink, or white flowers from which a **Bach flower remedy** can be prepared. This is said to have an anti-cancer effect. Clinical trials are at present under way.

olive

An evergreen tree from the Mediterranean area with small white flowers from which a **Bach flower remedy** can be prepared. This is said to help those people who are exhausted and drained of energy due to overwork, overexertion, or following an illness.

onion

A vegetable (*Allium cepa* of the lily family) with a globular or flask-shaped bulb. Onion contains cepenes — thiosulphates — which are responsible for the characteristic smell, and which have an antispasmodic effect that is useful in treating colic and relieving the bronchial constriction of asthma. Other constituents of onions reduce platelet aggregation and may have an anti-thrombotic effect, which may explain why traditionally onions are said to be good for the blood and for the heart. From early times the onion was widely used as a remedy for 'pestilence and plague', and cooked onions in various forms are still recommended to protect against colds and influenza. Onion juice can be used to treat insect bites and stings, and roasted onion can be applied externally to relieve earache.

opal
A form of silica which contains a large amount of water ('water stone'), and which is consequently fragile and regarded as unlucky by some people. It is usually white in colour, but the best gemstones have a rainbow effect. Fire opal is said to stimulate passion and the genital area, and to draw hidden emotions to the surface. It is recommended for helping women to relax during childbirth, and is also good for the lungs and to facilitate psychic awareness.
See also **crystal therapy**

ophthalmic somatology
See **iridology**

orange
A citrus fruit which is the source of several **aromatherapy** essential oils. The rind of *Citrus bergamia* is a source of *bergamot* oil, and *neroli* oil is prepared from the flowers. The edible sweet orange (*Citrus sinensis*) is a popular source of vitamin C, and the Seville orange (*Citrus aurantium*) is famous as the basis of **marmalade**. The colour orange balances the emotions and the digestive system, and is said to help reconcile people to their life and circumstances and release them from the past. Orange people are usually warm, sympathetic, and caring, but they show a tendency to self-pity and to undervalue themselves. Orange is associated with the spleen chakra.
See also **colour therapy**

orgone therapy
A therapeutic technique devised by Austrian psychoanalyst Wilhelm Reich (1897–1957) who set up a research centre in the USA at Orgonon in 1934. He claimed to have discovered a new form of universal energy, distinct from electromagnetism, which permeates everything and which he called 'Primordial or Cosmic Orgone Energy'. This energy is said to travel at the speed of light, and to be attracted by vegetable matter and reflected by metal. He designed *orgone accumulators*, boxes made of alternating layers of metal and wood

said to concentrate and store the energy, measured in units called *bions*, which is then supposedly available for healing purposes. He claimed that patients placed in boxes containing orgone accumulators could be cured of serious diseases including cancer. Dr Reich was investigated by the Federal Food and Drugs Administration in 1954, which denounced him as a charlatan, and he died in prison during a two-year jail sentence.

oriental diagnosis

A diagnostic technique typically originating in China, based on **traditional Chinese medicine**. Such techniques aim to identify disharmonies and imbalance in the body's energy, or blockages in the flow of **qi** through the meridian system. The system is based on the *eight principles*, the pillars of which are tongue and pulse diagnosis, and these form the basis upon which treatment by such techniques as **acupuncture, herbal medicine**, and **massage** can be devised.
See also **meridians**

Orr rebirthing

See **rebirthing**

orthomolecular medicine

[Greek *ortho* 'correct'] A term invented by Austrian chemist Linus Pauling (1901–) to describe the restoration and maintenance of good health by ensuring the correct levels of vitamins and minerals in the body.
See also **megavitamin therapy**

osteopathy

[Greek *osteo* 'bone'+*pathos* 'disease'] The diagnosis and treatment of pain and dysfunction in the musculo-skeletal system due to mechanical problems. The treatment involves **manipulation** to mobilize joints, free connective tissue restrictions, and consequently improve the blood flow to nerves and organs. The initial assessment usually includes a detailed history and physical examination, and may also involve laboratory and X-ray investigations. Treatment involves manipulation, stretching, and high velocity thrusts to correct any misalignments. Osteopathy is particularly popular for the treatment of backache and neck pain. In a more general sense, the term can refer to any bony structural abnormality which results in disease.

overuse syndrome
A common condition which presents as pain and loss of function of muscle and ligaments through excessive use; also called *repetitive strain injury*. It is seen particularly in musicians, sportsmen, and keyboard operators. Improvement can be achieved only by rest of the affected part.

P

paranormal therapy

Any method of healing which involves the use of spiritual or psychic forces for which there is as yet no scientific explanation, and in which all other possible explanations for the healing effect have been excluded. Examples include **absent healing, spiritual healing,** and **radiesthesia**.

pattern therapy

1 A system of treatment based on the belief that certain shapes and patterns (eg pyramids) concentrate the earth's electromagnetic or other energies. There are some supporting studies; for example, wounded mice may be shown to heal faster in spherical cages, and beer is said to taste different if stored in rectangular rather than spherical barrels.

2 The terms may also apply to the 'pattern' of dials on a **radionics** instrument, through which a healing pattern is said to be transmitted that stimulates a resonance in the patient's own healing energies. Homeopathic remedies are also said to have a 'healing energy pattern' imprinted on them.

See also **pyramid healing**

Paula Garburg system

A system of corrective exercises used in the treatment of postural problems and neuromuscular diseases such as polio, developed by Israeli physician Paula Garburg in Tel Aviv over the past 40 years. The exercises are designed to improve and strengthen the actions of the body's sphincters, thus allowing increased voluntary muscular control, and this is particularly helpful in some cases of urinary incontinence.

pearl

A gem, with a characteristic lustre, formed within bivalved molluscs, especially the pearl oyster. Pearls are associated with the moon and with water, and are said to be feminine and sympathetic in nature. They represent purity and chastity, and are reputed to heal damaged emotions and restore harmony.

peme /ˈpiːmiː/

An abbreviation of **Pulsed Electro Magnetic Energy**, generated by an electrical machine and directed at damaged tissues in order to recharge them with electromagnetic energy. The technique is claimed to accelerate normal healing processes by up to 50%.
See also **magnetic therapy**

Pen Chiao

[Chinese, 'Great Herbal'] A classical text of **traditional Chinese medicine**, a multi-authored document attributed to Shen Nung and thought to date from around 3000 BC. It lists 365 herbs and their properties, as well as describing other treatment methods such as **acupuncture, moxibustion, massage**, exercises, and surgery.

peridot

A gem quality crystal of olivine (*chrysolite*), which is an iron silicate, brilliant yellow-green in colour. It is especially associated with the spleen **chakra**. Peridot clears emotional congestion, and is regarded as good for both the mind and the liver, aiding the absorption and digestion of food.
See also **crystal therapy**

personal construct therapy

A system of psychotherapy proposed by George Kelly in 1955, which is characterized by:

1 *enactment*, which is a kind of role-play between the therapist and patient, acting out difficult situations;

2 *self-characterization*, in which patients are asked to write a biography of themselves as they think they would be seen by a close friend;

3 *fixed role technique*, where patients pretend to be a fictional character created by the therapist in order to illustrate how other people react to them; patients are thus led to review their own personal behaviour;

4 *repertory grid analysis*, which involves filling out a questionnaire designed to discover how patients view themselves and the world about them.

personality

The patterns of thought and behaviour which characterize each individual. Personality traits can be genetically determined, but there is a substantial contribution from 'learned behaviour' through which the environment and major influences such as the parents affect personality development. Some recognizable personality types show consistent predisposition to both mental and physical illnesses; for example, 'Type A' personalities ('achievers' constantly striving for success, and to attain self-imposed goals which maintain high stress levels), whilst apparently having enhanced resistance to minor disorders, show an increased susceptibility to coronary artery disease.

perverse energy

A concept in **traditional Chinese medicine** which encompasses all the various factors causing disease. The Chinese character *xie qi* consists partly of the ideogram for 'canine tooth' or 'something which attacks', and implies the intrusion of a disturbance of the body's normal energy balance. Perverse energy can refer to external environmental factors which can invade the body (eg wind, heat, damp, cold, dryness) or internal factors where the emotions can interfere with the flow of **qi** and blood, causing dysfunction in the internal organs (eg joy, anger, pensiveness, grief.)

pfaffia

A plant of the family *Aramanthaceae* (*Pfaffia paniculata*) which flourishes in tropical Brazil. It contains a wide variety of

nutrients, as well as active constituents such as pfaffic acid
and various pfaffosides. These have been shown to give some
benefit in cardiovascular and degenerative disease, improve
pancreatic function, correct hormone imbalances, and inhibit
tumour growth.

phenomenological psychotherapy
See **humanistic psychotherapy**

physiatrics
A form of natural therapy from the Chinese system of **qi gong**.
This uses a machine invented by a Chinese biomedical
engineer, Zhou Lin, which is said to stimulate the resonance
of the body tissues and regulate the body's bioelectric field.
This is claimed to accelerate healing and pain relief.

physical rhythm
A rhythm which controls the muscular and physical systems
of the body, and affects strength, confidence, stamina, and
drive. When in a positive phase, the body's powers of
endurance and strength are at its best, but when in a negative
phase, people feel tired and lethargic, and lack confidence
and enthusiasm.
See also **biorhythms**

physiotherapy
A widely accepted and respected form of complementary
medical treatment which uses physical methods to treat
muscular and skeletal problems. The methods employed by
physiotherapists are usually well-established and well-
studied, and include active and passive exercises which may
be specific (eg to treat back pain or mobilize joints) or general
(to improve a patient's general level of fitness and mobility).
Many physiotherapists employ machines such as ultrasound,
short-wave diathermy, and **TENS**, to relieve pain and
accelerate healing processes. They may also perform massage, acupuncture, or other methods of treatment according
to their personal interests and training.

phytotherapy

phytotherapy

[Greek *phyton* 'plant'+*therapeuein* 'to heal'] An alternative title for **herbal medicine**, widely known on the Continent (but less used in the UK). It refers to the study of plants and the use of plant-based medicines for healing purposes. Most phytotherapists are conventional doctors who also use herbal remedies and who generally believe that using whole plants is a safer and more effective way of giving treatment than isolating and using purified ingredients. The remedies are generally less concentrated than orthodox medicines, and are claimed to work in a more balanced way and to cause fewer side effects.

Pilate's technique

An exercise technique developed from the training routines of athletes and dancers which emphasizes the control of both movement and breathing. 'Realignment exercises' are practised, which are said to concentrate the body and mind and to result in improved posture, with consequent reduction in tension, fatigue, and stress.

pine

An evergreen conifer of the family *Pinaceae* which produces a fragrant resin and from the leaves of which a **Bach flower remedy** can be prepared. It is said to help those who have feelings of guilt about past events, or who blame themselves even when they have done nothing wrong.

pineal gland

A small gland situated above the third ventricle deep in the brain, which secretes hormones including melatonin, serotonin, and betacarboline. It works in conjunction with the pituitary gland in controlling other hormones and body systems, and is itself under feedback from other glands, such as the thyroid. It is regarded as the seat of second sight, or as the 'third eye' which corresponds to the **ajna** chakra (sixth chakra), regarded as the site of psychic activities including telepathy.
See also **chakra**

pineapple

An evergreen plant from South America (*Ananas comosus*) cultivated for its fleshy yellow fruit. Pineapple juice is rich in vitamins A and B, and both stems and fruit contain a mixture of enzymes called *bromelain* which has been used as a traditional remedy for inflammation and burns for centuries. More recently bromelain has been thought to have anti-cancer properties, after an inhibitory effect was demonstrated on leukaemia cells growing in a culture system.

pinhole glasses

Spectacles with lenses not made of glass, but which consist of an opaque sheet, usually made of plastic, with many perforations through which light passes to the eye. This is said to give improvement in vision for patients suffering from a wide variety of visual defects, including shortsightedness, longsightedness, astigmatism, and eye strain. The beneficial effect of the pinholes is said to be the result of reducing the overall amount of light reaching the eye, thus reducing the effective aperture of the eye, which makes focusing easier. These glasses are used to exercise the eyes for those patients with focusing problems, and may improve brain to eye coordination, allowing improved focusing without the need for conventional glasses.

PK

See **psychokinesis**

placebo effect /pləˈsiːboʊ/

A beneficial effect produced by suggestion and expectation, in the absence of an active treatment agent. The extent of this effect is particularly influenced by the patient-therapist relationship, and is said to be most marked with 'dramatic' forms of intervention such as those requiring complicated apparatus or highly coloured medicines. In this situation, approximately 30% of patients will report subjective improvement with any therapy that is offered.

plum blossom needle

An **acupuncture** device consisting of five or seven needles mounted in a bundle on a handle rather like a small hammer.

The needles are evenly spaced, the tips are on the same level, and the device is used by tapping vertically on to the skin surface with a movement of the wrist. Light tapping results in superficial redness and heavy tapping may cause bleeding. Tapping may be applied to an affected area, eg along the sides of the spinal column, on particular acupuncture points, or along the course of **meridians**.

PNI
See **psychoneuroimmunology**

podiatry
See **chiropody**

polarity therapy
A system of treatment developed by Randolph Stone (1890–1983), who studied **osteopathy, naturopathy**, and **chiropractic**, and used exercise, **massage**, and **manipulation** to stimulate, release, and balance the 'life energy' in the body. He taught that the body has five energy centres corresponding to the **five elements** (earth, water, fire, air, ether), and that most illnesses are caused by blockage of the flow of energy between these centres as a result of bad living or bad environment. Good health depends on the free and uninterrupted flow of vital energy throughout the body, and the therapy aims to remove any blockages and to discover the 'energy' cause of any illness. The components of treatment are:

1 polarity energy balancing through touch manipulation;
2 polarity yoga exercises involving rocking and stretching postures with vocal expressions to release and encourage movement of the body's energy;
3 dietary changes which may involve a cleansing programme to expel toxins, and then dietary advice to maintain healthy eating;
4 counselling to develop self-awareness and positive thoughts and attitudes to the body and to life in general.

postural integration

A system of therapy designed to realign the posture and hence restore natural energy flow through the body. This results in a change of physical, mental, and emotional patterns. Physical and emotional stress and trauma cause tension and loss of flexibility in both muscles and connective tissue, which results in pain and unbalanced posture. The therapist may use a variety of techniques, including **massage**, movement, **rolfing**, and **acupressure** to realign the posture.

post-viral fatigue syndrome

See **myalgic encephalomyelitis**

potato

A tuber-producing plant (*Solanum tuberosum* of the family *Solanaceae*), the fruits of which are poisonous when green and uncooked, but which is popular worldwide as a vegetable. Potatoes and potato water (after boiling) are used in treating rheumatic pains, warts, and chapped hands. Raw potato can be used as a plaster and a burns dressing. Rubbing with a raw potato is said to relieve the pain of chilblains. Eating the green fruit of potatoes is hazardous because of high levels of alkaloids, and more than 2 000 cases of alkaloid poisoning due to potatoes have been documented, some of them fatal.

potentization

The process by which a homeopathic remedy is prepared and becomes more powerful as it is serially diluted. Homeopathic remedies are not active in the chemical sense of drug activity. Theoretically if a remedy is diluted to more than 10^{-24} (12 C), there can be no original molecules of the substance left in the preparation (Avogadro's law), but the remedy is said to 'imprint' itself on the diluent (ie water molecules). Since the energy is said to be enhanced by each dilution, the homeopathic remedy has a high intrinsic energy which can in turn stimulate the body's own bioenergetic system and possibly even 'imprint' on it to produce a self-replicating effect.

prenatal therapy

In preparing a homeopathic remedy, plants are collected in the growing state, crushed, and an alcoholic extract made by soaking and filtering, known as the 'Mother Tincture'. This is diluted with alcohol to 1 part in 10 or 1 part in 100, and then shaken or succussed by hand or machine. One drop of this solution is then transferred to the next phial which contains 9 or 99 drops of diluent, and further **succussion** performed. Each stage of dilution is designated either 1 D (decimal) or 1 C (centesimal), which defines the 'potency' of the preparation. Commonly used potencies are 6 C, 12 C, 30 C, 200 C, 1 M, and 10 M.

See also **homeopathy; trituration**

prenatal therapy

A gentle manipulation of the spinal reflex areas of the hands, feet, and head, with the aim of releasing energy blockages which may have developed during gestation.

See also **metamorphic technique**

primal therapy

A therapeutic technique devised by American psychiatrist Arthur Janov, who believed that childhood trauma, emotional difficulties, and lack of affection can lead to nervous and emotional problems as an adult. He developed primal therapy to help the adult patient express and come to terms with these feelings — a process that he described by the expression 'voicing the primal scream'. Janov's work has been available in the UK since 1976, and has been popularized by many books and famous patients (eg John Lennon).

probiotics

Treatment by the ingestion of 'friendly' bacteria (eg *lactobacilli*) which work with the patient's own gut flora to encourage a balance between the harmless bacteria which live there and the putrefactive bacteria, yeasts, and fungi which may be causing illness by their presence. A contrast may be drawn with *antibiotics*, which are intended to suppress or kill bacteria.

See also **dysbiosis**

propolis /'prɒpəlɪs/
A substance used by bees to seal the hive against attacks by bacteria and viruses. It contains a wide variety of complex substances, and is one of the richest known sources of bioflavonoids. Propolis is often recommended as a dietary supplement by beauticians and nutritionists.

proving
[German *prüfung* 'test, trial'] A term used by German physician Samuel Hahnemann (1755–1843), who developed the basis of **homeopathy** by testing medicinal substances on himself, his family, and his friends. He administered tiny doses of the substances over periods of weeks or months, and observed the symptoms they produced.

psionic medicine /(p)saɪˈɒnɪk/
[Greek *psion* 'psychic'] A system which combines orthodox medicine with **radiesthesia**, devised by Dr George Laurence, who founded the Psionic Medical Society in 1968. The system involves using paranormal faculties which require intuitive ability to examine 'witnesses' such as blood and hair samples, as well as employing normal diagnostic techniques such as taking a detailed medical history. The diagnosis emphasizes predisposing causes, rather than being directly related to physical symptoms and illnesses, which are seen as a disturbance of the 'vital balance'. Imbalances can be detected and treated homeopathically before major symptoms become established, by using a pendulum and special charts. This system is said to be useful in treating chronic and otherwise incurable conditions.
See also **homeopathy**

psi powers /(p)saɪ/
[Greek *psion* 'psychic'] A term introduced by British psychologist R H Thouless for phenomena which cannot be explained without assuming the presence of paranormal forces. Since these appear inconsistently, reproducible experiments to demonstrate their effect have proved

extremely difficult to organize. The powers include extrasensory perception, **psychokinesis, telepathy**, precognition, **clairvoyance**, and **psychometry**, any of which may explain the actions and effects of 'healers' in some instances.

psychic counselling

[Greek *psyche* 'soul'] A method of counselling in which the counsellor uses a person's own **aura** to gather information which will allow the patient to understand his or her own problems and difficulties, to develop insight, and to decide upon the best course of action. The counsellor encourages patients to make their own choices and decisions, but there may sometimes be an overlap with *psychic healing*, whereby the healer may transfer to the recipients the energy they need to heal themselves.

psychic surgery

A dramatic form of treatment particularly associated with the Espiritista Church in the Philippines. The healers or 'surgeons' are said to act as channels for the Archangel Michael (or occasionally the Virgin Mary) and 'operate' upon patients by moving their hands over the afflicted part. This usually results in the appearance of blood and possibly pieces of viscera or tumour, but no cut or scar is present after the procedure. There have been some dramatic anecdotal accounts of the results of such procedures which have not, however, been subject to any rigorous scrutiny.

psychoanalysis

The psychotherapeutic approach to mental illness and emotional problems, pioneered by Austrian psychoanalyst Sigmund Freud (1856–1939), who attempted to explain behaviour in terms of the interplay between the unconscious and conscious mind. He believed that primitive instincts, particularly concerning sex, and painful memories may be banished into the unconscious mind but then revealed in dreams, in creative activities such as writing and painting, and sometimes in the form of overt psychiatric illness. The process of analysis enables the person to confront these repressed feelings, and thereby release the tension between the conscious and subconscious which may result in a modification of personality.

See also **psychotherapy**

psychodrama

A form of group therapy which developed from an idea by Austrian psychiatrist Jacob Moreno, a contemporary of Sigmund Freud, in which groups of people take it in turns to act out each other's real-life situations and problems. Strong emotions can be generated during these sessions, and the therapist may use these emotions to interpret situations and to help participants come to terms with their own feelings and learn new ways of dealing with their problems.

psychokinesis *or* PK

[Greek *psyche* 'soul' + *kinesis* 'motion'] A paranormal phenomenon, defined as the means by which the mind directly influences matter without physical manipulation or in ways which can be understood by physical science.

See also **paranormal therapy**

psychology

The scientific study of human behaviour. Psychologists are employed usually as industrial, educational, experimental, social, or clinical psychologists. It is only the latter group that deal with emotional and behavioural problems, and who have experience in applied psychology in the form of **psychotherapy**.

psychometry

A form of parapsychology which refers to the process by which information can be derived directly from an object without any sensory cues being present. The information usually relates to past events associated with the object or its owner.

psychoneuroimmunology (PNI)

An emerging discipline which emphasizes the fundamental links between psychology, neurophysiology, and immunology. All neuroendocrine hormones and neuropeptides (eg adrenaline, serotonin, endorphins) have effects on the immune system, and immunological transmitter substances (eg lymphokines) have effects on other parts of the body, including the nervous system.

psychosomatic medicine
[Greek *psyche* 'soul'+*soma* 'body'] The study of the inter-dependence and interaction of psychological and physical factors in producing illness. Emotions such as anger, grief, and jealousy can cause stress, which leads to sustained hyperactivity of the sympathetic nervous system, release of adrenaline and other hormones into the blood stream, and consequent adverse effects on their target organs. The clinical problems which commonly result include headaches, hypertension, and stomach ulcers.

psychosynthesis
A principle developed by Italian psychiatrist Roberto Assagioli (1888–1974), who believed that all people have the potential to develop a balanced personality and to make the best of themselves, and should be made aware of their own responsibility for personal self-development. This form of psychotherapy aims to provide support and guidance so that individuals can realize their full potential for good health and good interpersonal relationships. This process is intended to transform, balance, and integrate various aspects of the personality, and to help subjects to apply their minds to achieving maximum potential in both work and personal life.

psychotherapy
A therapeutic approach which aims to explain people's behaviour patterns and to provide guidelines for treating emotional problems. There are hundreds of different schools of psychotherapy, but they share the goal of enabling patients to understand themselves and their feelings and relationships with others, and to explore new patterns of behaviour which may help them deal with their emotional problems. The main approaches are psychoanalytic, humanistic, cognitive, and behavioural. Some psychotherapists are clinical psychologists, but the title is not yet regulated by law

in the UK, and there is no licensing procedure or formal requirement for qualifications. Practitioners come from a variety of backgrounds, including psychiatry, psychology, social work, teaching, and management.
See also **psychoanalysis**

pulse diagnosis

One of the 'pillars' of diagnosis in **traditional Chinese medicine**. TCM texts describe 18 pulses, nine on each radial artery at the wrist (although pulses are also felt at the neck and legs). Each radial pulse is palpated at three positions and three different depths. Each of the major organs (**zang fu**) is represented in the pulses, and the characteristics of the pulses allow diagnosis of individual organ pathology. The pulse rate is assessed against the patient's breathing rate, but there are also variations in rhythm and 'shape' of the pulse, and 28 different 'qualities' are described (eg rapid, slippery, tight, empty, stagnant) which have associations with particular patterns of dysharmony.
See also **pulsograph**

pulsograph

An apparatus for demonstrating the characteristics of the radial pulse, recorded by a piezo-electric pressure sensor and analysed using a six-channel oscilloscope. The pattern of the pulse is then interpreted closely following the principles of **traditional Chinese medicine**.
See also **pulse diagnosis**

pyramid healing

An approach to healing which relies on the beneficial effects associated with the shape of a pyramid. For example, sleeping beneath a pyramid is said to give more refreshing sleep, and there are also anecdotal reports of women recording alteration in menstrual period and relief from dysmenorrhoea. Pyramids are said to enhance plant growth, and have been used for storing fruit and vegetables. It has been suggested that a pyramidal configuration, which reproduces the exact proportions of the Great Pyramids, where the height X is the radius of a circle whose circumference Y is the same as the circumference of the square base Z of the pyramid, may in some way concentrate electromagnetic energy, or affect the balance of positive and negative ions in the air contained within it.

See also **pattern therapy**

Q

qi /ʧiː/
A term used in **traditional Chinese medicine**, also written as *chi*, which originally meant air, breath or energy, and later assumed the meaning of 'vital essence', the supreme nourishing and protecting energy in the body, which circulates through the **acupuncture meridians**. The circulation of qi may be stimulated by the breathing exercises known as **qi gong** and the martial art **tai chi chuan**. Various forms of qi are described, such as that derived from food (*gu qi*) and air (*ta qi*), and the qi received from one's parents known as 'before heaven' or pre-natal qi, which is gradually used up during life and only partly replaced by *gu qi* and *ta qi*.

qi gong

[Chinese *qi* 'energy', 'the air' + *gong* 'time, practice'] A Chinese system of physical exercises, breathing, and mental training which has the aim of strengthening the body's internal energy and controlling the circulation of the vital **qi**. The various systems of exercise share fundamental principles:

1 adjustment of the body, encouraging relaxation to allow the qi to flow through the **meridians**;
2 adjustment of the mind, which means maintaining concentration and focusing the attention;
3 adjustment of the breath.

Various types of qi gong are described, broadly divided into static and moving, and hard and soft. Specific exercises have been developed to maintain health and encourage healing, and other forms are used in martial arts and for spiritual development.

Quackbusters

See **Healthwatch**

quartz

A crystallized form of silicone dioxide which may be clear, white, or translucent. It includes some semi-precious stones which may be coloured, such as amethyst.

See also **crystal therapy; rose quartz; smoky quartz**

quantic theory

A holistic approach to diagnosis which assumes that all aspects of a health problem are of equal importance. The electrical, spiritual, psychological, and environmental characteristics of the body are believed to be integrated together and to function in a logical fashion. These can be tested holistically by the **eclosion** computer to derive a working diagnosis from which to formulate a treatment plan.

See also **eclosion system; holism**

R

radiance technique

A system of therapy derived from Tibetan teachings. Its aim is to balance the chakras and harmonize the mind, body, and spirit in order to promote relaxation, encourage natural healing abilities, and make effective use of the body's energy in daily life.

See also **chakra**

radiesthesia

The use of **dowsing** both to diagnose disease and to select a suitable remedy (which is usually herbal or homeopathic). This system was developed in France at the beginning of this century by the Abbés Bouley and Mermet. It was introduced to the UK in 1939 by British surgeon George Laurence, who founded the Medical Society for the Study of Radiesthesia. The practitioner uses a pendulum to examine a sample ('witness') supplied by the patient, which is usually hair, nail clippings, blood, or saliva. The pendulum swings over the witness as questions are posed by the dowser, and diagnosis is made by comparing the response with reference samples taken from various diseases, using a specially designed diagnostic rule or triangle.

See also **radionics**

radio-allergic solvents test (RAST)

A blood test in which a radio-immuno assay (ie one using radio isotopes) is used to demonstrate the immunoglobulin response to food extracts, and thus to establish whether an allergy is truly present; also called **radio-allergy absorbent test**.

radionics

The practice of **radiesthesia**, using an instrument to diagnose disease in human beings, animals, and plants, and then to treat the disease at a distance using radiesthesic principles. The initial 'black box' was produced by American neurologist Albert Abrams (d. 1924). This device, which contained no electronic circuitry or power source, depended upon the diseased tissue or 'witness' radiating abnormal waves of some kind. An American chiropractor, Ruth Drowns, continued Abrams' work, but was investigated and prosecuted by the American Federal Food and Drugs Administration in 1951, being convicted of fraud and medical quackery. Work has continued in England with British engineer George De La Warr, who formed the Radionic and Magnetic Centre organization in 1965. A sample of hair, blood, or nail clippings from a patient is said to produce energy waves to which the radionics instrument can be tuned by rotating a small magnet. There is a series of dials on the instrument with frequency settings corresponding to various disease conditions. The operator takes a written list of the patient's symptoms, and then uses a pendulum or rubber diaphragm to analyse the person's physical, mental, and spiritual state to determine the cause of any disharmony. The treatment plan will probably involve broadcasting healing waves with the radionics instrument, but may also include counselling, dietary advice, and other forms of treatment according to the particular interests of the practitioner.

radon

Element number 86, a colourless, odourless, radioactive gas (liquid boiling-point $-62°C$) produced by the decay of radium in rock (usually granite). There are several isotopes, the longest (Rn^{222}) of which has a half-life of four days. Some areas, particularly situated on granite, have high levels of radon exposure (measured in becquerels) and the gas can penetrate buildings through the floors and walls, leading to a dangerous build-up in concentration unless these are well sealed and there is adequate ventilation. Radon can accumulate in the lungs, causing respiratory damage including lung cancer. However, exposure to radon in underground caverns has been used as a form of treatment in Germany.
See also **becquerel**

rainbow healing

A healing technique based on the principle that water placed in coloured containers and then exposed to sunlight supposedly takes on the intrinsic energy of the colour of the container. This water is then drunk by patients deficient in the colour to restore balance.

See also **colour therapy**

RAST

See **radio-allergic solvents test**

raw food diet

A diet in which at least 80% of the food (by weight) is eaten raw, mainly as fruit and vegetables. The human digestive tract is similar to that of plant-eating animals, and is not designed for a high meat diet. Raw food avoids losing vitamins, minerals, and enzymes through the process of cooking, and also tends to be alkaline, which reduces the amount of acid in the diet.

rebirthing

A form of **psychotherapy** in which the patient undergoes regression to birth, so that negative thoughts and attitudes which might have resulted from traumatic experiences at birth can be changed by reliving the experience. There are various forms of rebirthing practised, such as *Orr rebirthing*, which involves the use of regular breathing; *water rebirthing*, which may involve being submerged in a bath of water with or without a snorkel; and *group rebirthing*, in which the patient who is to be reborn is enclosed in a 'womb' constructed of other members of the group, who sit and press against the person, using cushions as buffers.

receptive crystal

A crystal with a seven-sided flat face which can be used to draw out pain or perverse energy and is also said to stimulate the capacity to listen to our own inner wisdom and to be able to record and store memories of meditation.

See also **crystal therapy**

recommended daily amount (RDA)

The recommended minimal daily requirement of essential nutrients, such as vitamins and trace elements, which need to be consumed to avoid the effects of deficiency.

red

A strong physical colour which represents the fire element, suggesting heat, action, and innovation. Red personalities tend to be leaders and adventurers, but may be aggressive and insensitive. Red is associated with the base **chakra**, which represents reproduction and sexual activity.

reflexology

A Chinese and Indian system of diagnosis and treatment dating from 3000 BC, often used together with **acupuncture**. It is based on the belief that the whole body is represented on the foot (mostly on the soles of the feet), and that the internal organs can be stimulated by pressing particular areas of the foot (less commonly the hands). The reflexology zones do not correspond exactly to either the nervous system or acupuncture **meridians**, but the same principles of illness due to 'blockage' of energy channels is applied as in **traditional Chinese medicine**. The method was first used in the West in 1913 by William Fitzgerald, an ENT surgeon interested in acupuncture. Reflexology involves palpation to locate sites of tenderness, or crystalline deposits beneath the skin, which are taken to represent remote organ disease. Treatment is by pressure and deep massage, and is most successful for functional disorders such as constipation, headaches, and stress states. Reflexology is not effective in treating structural abnormalities or surgical problems.

reflex zone therapy

An ancient form of healing practised by the Chinese and Egyptians, dating from 3000 BC. **Massage** of reflex points which relate to corresponding areas of the body, such as the **reflexology** zones, restores and balances the flow of **qi**.

regression

A psychological defence mechanism by which a person assumes a behaviour pattern appropriate to a younger age. *Past-life regression* is a form of **psychotherapy** which aims to establish contact with supposed previous incarnations in order to understand what **karmic** lessons were learnt during those lives and thus to employ all the wisdom and experience gained in this present life.

See also **reincarnation**

Reichian therapy

A system of treatment developed by Austrian psychoanalyst Wilhelm Reich (1897–1957). He taught that unpleasant experiences and feelings in the unconscious mind can create both psychological problems and physical tension ('body armouring'). Physical manipulation to relax this body armouring releases tension and frees repressed emotions. Psychological and other problems result from a blockage of orgone energy.

See also **orgone therapy**

reincarnation

The belief, found chiefly in Eastern cultures such as Buddhism and Hinduism, that the spirit survives in an afterlife and can then return again to earth to live in another body. There are numerous cases of previous life memories recorded particularly with the help of techniques such as hypnotic regression. Evidence cited in support of the theory of reincarnation includes the phenomenon of *xenoglossia* — the speaking of a language which has not been learnt by the person in their present life.

See also **regression**

reiki /'raɪki/

[Japanese, 'universal energy'] A system of natural healing developed by Japanese theologian Mikao Usui in the 19th century based on Sanskrit sutras believed to relate to cosmic symbols used by the Buddha for healing. Healing energy is channelled into the patient by laying on of hands to activate the body's natural healing processes and restore harmony.

reinforcement

A technique of **behavioural therapy** developed by American psychologist Burrhus Skinner (1904–90), who encouraged animals and people to take an active part in learning. A system of rewards (pleasant experiences) is used for behaviour to be encouraged, and punishment (unpleasant experiences) for unwanted behaviour.

relaxation

A technique used to combat stress. Human beings can cope with brief periods of stress (eg in response to danger) in which the nervous system is overactive and the muscles stimulated more than usual. Prolonged states of arousal result in illness, which can include anxiety, headaches, and hypertension. Regular relaxation is essential to combat stress. *Passive relaxation*, such as resting and listening to music, allows the muscles to relax; *active relaxation*, which may include exercising to relieve tension and performing meditation techniques, encourages both muscular and mental calmness.

relaxation meter

See **biofeedback** and **electrical skin resistance**

repetitive strain injury

See **overuse syndrome**

rescue remedy

A compound remedy which includes five of the 38 **Bach flower remedies**:

1 star of Bethlehem for shock;
2 rock rose for fear and panic;
3 Impatiens for mental and physical tension;
4 cherry plum for loss of emotional control;
5 clematis for the distant feeling which precedes a faint.

This remedy is recommended for emergency situations when there is panic, shock, or stress. It is said to restore calmness and allow the body's healing energies to work.

resonance therapy

A system of therapy developed at the Institute for Advanced Health Research in Yeovil, Somerset, which regards each disease symptom as part of a sequence of body malfunctions for which there is a mathematical solution, or 'resonance'. This can be calculated for each symptom, using expressions based on the connection between the illness and environmental stresses. Bioelectric tests can identify disorders and the means of correcting them. All forms of therapy, including lights, flowers, foods, colours, essential oils, and crystals, are deemed to act by introducing healing resonances into the organs where they are needed.

An *Environmental Stress Eliminator* is a resonance generator which can be tuned in to eliminate any environmental stresses within its area of influence.

rock rose

A small evergreen shrub with white, yellow, or red flowers from which a **Bach flower remedy** may be prepared. This is said to help those who suffer panic and terror attacks, whether these have a rational basis or not.

rock water

Pure water taken from a natural well which is exposed to sunlight, and which can be used (like holy water) to bring peace and understanding. This is listed as a **Bach flower remedy** to help those who suffer from tension and self-reproach as a result of imposing unreasonable and rigid standards upon themselves and others.

Rogerian counselling

A counselling technique devised by American therapist Carl Rogers (1902–87). He listed the three basic requirements of a therapist if a client is to benefit from psychotherapy:

1 the therapist must have empathy, ie the ability to see the world through the client's eyes (and this must be realized by the client);
2 the therapist must be genuine and have the real understanding that comes from having personally undergone therapy;

3 the therapist must show warmth and make the client feel valued and supported.

The client's own point of view is of primary importance, and therapists should be trained to listen and respond in an empathetic way so as to encourage clients to work out their own solutions to their problems, rather than having the therapist's views thrust upon them.

rolfing

A system of deep massage, developed by American biological chemist Dr Ida Rolf (1896–1979), which manipulates soft tissues to break down any abnormal connective tissue formed as a result of abnormal posture or muscular contraction. Her system of 'structural integration' is said to loosen up the body and allow realignment and readjustment over the course of ten one-hour treatment sessions. The patient is first photographed from the back, front, and sides to help detect and demonstrate abnormal posture and tension. The therapist's own body weight is used through elbows, knuckles, hands, and fingers to apply pressure, with the object of realigning physical structures in a straight vertical line so that the earth's gravity can give proper support to the body's own energy fields. Some subjects report pain and discomfort during treatment, but may be up to half an inch taller by the end.

rose quartz

Quartz of a delicate pink colour, said to be feminine, gentle, and soothing and to help cure aches, pains, phobias, vulnerability, and inadequacy. It is also reputed to be good for the complexion, smoothing wrinkles, and even for healing a broken heart!

royal jelly

A substance produced by the salivary glands of worker bees to nourish the queen bee and the larvae that are destined to become queens. It contains approximately 20 amino acids, some of which are essential for human beings, and also vitamins including vitamin B complex and vitamin C, with trace elements including potassium, chromium, manganese, and nickel. There are many anecdotal claims of its beneficial effects as a high-energy food and when taken orally for ME, rheumatoid arthritis, and cardiovascular disease. It is also included as an ingredient in various skin creams and lotions which are claimed to have a rejuvenating effect.

ruby

A red gemstone form of corundum, found mostly in Burma, Sri Lanka, and Thailand, which is said to be the 'king of gems' and a powerful stone of the spirit. It energizes the heart, stimulates the will to live, and symbolizes lasting love, marriage, and loyalty.
See also **crystal therapy**

rutilated quartz

A clear quartz, containing small veins of gold or silver formed from titanium oxide, which is said to focus and direct the mind. The crystal holds connecting links with both past and future, friends, and family.
See also **crystal therapy**

S

SAD
See **seasonal affective disorder**

sahasra
The seventh **chakra**, situated at the crown of the head.

salicylates
Naturally-occurring salts in fruits and vegetables such as cucumber, tomatoes, berries, apples, and oranges. Synthetic salicylates are also used to flavour sweets, ice creams, soft drinks, and cake mixtures. This group of substances include aspirin, which was first prepared from willow bark, and is widely used as an analgesic and anti-inflammatory agent. There is chemical similarity to tartrazine, which is used as a food additive.

salt-free diet
A diet which is as free from salt as possible, and which is particularly recommended for patients with cardiovascular and kidney disorders. It is very difficult to achieve completely salt-free food, because salt is naturally occurring and widely used in food manufacture and processing. A high salt intake has been shown to be associated with hypertension.

sapphire
A gemstone variety of corundum, which may be coloured deep blue by ferric iron or titanium, or coloured pink, green, or yellow by other minerals. It is said to represent wisdom, beauty, and truth, to be associated with heavenly virtue, devotion, and self-control, and to assist with the healing of infections. The *star sapphire* is the stone of destiny, which is reputed to make dreams come true.
See also **crystal therapy**

sauna

A form of steam bath, originating in Scandinavia, in which steam is generated by splashing water on heated stones or a stove, usually in an insulated pine cabin. The heat and humidity in the cabin induce sweating, which eliminates waste and toxins through the skin as well as stimulating the circulation. The temperature is usually maintained at 28–38°C but must not rise above 43°C. The sauna bath is sometimes combined with light beating with birch leaves to further stimulate the circulation.

scleranthus

A small plant (*Scleranthus annuus*) with tangled stems and green flowers, growing on sandy soil, particularly on uncultivated land where there is natural grazing. A **Bach flower remedy** can be prepared from the flowering heads which is said to help those suffering with emotional distress resulting from indecision and rapid swings of mood.

sea bands

Elasticated bands with a plastic stud, worn around the wrists to apply pressure to the **acupuncture** point Pericardium 6. This point is used for treating nausea and vomiting, including that due to travel sickness and pregnancy.

seasonal affective disorder (SAD)

A form of winter depression which may affect as many as 5–10% of the population. Sufferers complain of symptoms of depression, including extreme fatigue, increased desire to sleep, and increased appetite, particularly for carbohydrates, which leads to weight gain and lethargy. Light enters the body through the eyes where, as well as stimulating light receptors to produce vision, it also affects the pineal gland, through which hormonal and neurochemical messengers are released that influence the body's biological rhythms. Light also induces the formation of vitamin D in the skin. The best cure for SAD is natural sunlight, but it is possible to simulate sunlight using an artificial light box which emits light at around 2500 lux, the minimum intensity necessary to

influence hormonal mechanisms (indoor lighting usually emits around 500 lux). Sitting for four to six hours per day in front of a light box will relieve symptoms within five days in 80% of patients.
See also **light therapy**

selenium

A metalloid element (number 34) used in photo-electric cells to convert light energy to electricity and also in rectifiers to convert alternating to direct current. The mineral selenium is sometimes used as a food supplement, usually in the form of brewer's yeast, and is said to enhance immune responses and possibly to affect white blood cell production, thereby increasing resistance to infection. Selenium is a component of the enzyme glutathione perioxidase, which protects cells from oxidative damage. It may also be used to treat dandruff and ringworm in preparations which contain selenium sulphide.

sensitivity

An adverse reaction of the body to a noxious stimulus. This is usually in the form of a chemical or food substance, but it may also be a physical agent, such as heat, cold, or sunlight.

sensitivity training

A form of **psychotherapy** intended to build better relationships by exploring people's interactions with each other, making them more aware of their own feelings and encouraging them to relate to each other more truthfully.

sensory resonance

A 'total sensory experience' in which electronic circuitry converts music to auditory, visual, and tactile stimuli. This is said, by the manufacturer of the apparatus, to turn off the brain's analytical function, so that the user can 'experience consciousness directly rather than conceptualizing it', although how these electronically generated sensations can accomplish this is not clear.
See also **vibrasound**

sex therapy

A form of therapy popularized through the works of American sexologists William Masters (1915–) and Virginia Johnson (1925–) first published in 1966, which aims to provide short-term support for couples with a range of sexual difficulties such as impotence, vaginismus, and orgasmic problems. It is essential that there is an initial medical history and assessment to eliminate organic disease, following which both male and female therapists usually work with the couple, beginning by encouraging them to touch each other in a non-sexual way and abstain from intercourse and then working through a graduated programme, emphasizing the need for mutual communication and understanding, which addresses the couple's particular problems and culminates in free sex.

shamanism

Any religion based on the mediating power of a shaman, who is a person believed to possess special powers of communication with spirits who help to diagnose and cure illness, or advise about other problems. Shamanism emphasizes harmony and balance in the universe, and the practice of the 'way of the four directions' which involves (*a*) honouring the four kingdoms of animal, plant, mineral, and human; (*b*) honouring the four elements of earth, air, fire, and water; and (*c*) honouring the four aspects of humanity, which are mental, physical, emotional, and spiritual.

sheng cycle

In **traditional Chinese medicine,** the 'generating' sequence, in which each element is generated by its predecessor and in turn generates its successor. Thus: wood generates fire; fire generates earth; earth generates metal; metal generates water; and water generates wood. Because of the association of the elements with the internal organs, the sheng cycle can be used as a basis for interpreting disease (patterns of disharmony) and formulating treatment.
See also **five elements**

shen tao

A form of **acupressure** based on the use of the 'eight extra **meridians**', using light finger pressure on **acupuncture** points to regulate and balance the **qi**. This in turn promotes the body's natural healing abilities. Some believe shen tao to be the 'mother of acupuncture'.

shiatsu

[Japanese, 'finger pressure'] A form of **massage** using pressure from fingers, thumbs, and sometimes elbows, knees, hands, and feet applied to **acupuncture** points and **meridians** either as firm massage to stimulate energy flow, or to specific points to release and balance the flow of energy. Healing energy may be transmitted from the practitioner through shiatsu massage, and regular treatment may be used to prevent disease and maintain a harmonic energy balance. Diagnosis is based on **traditional Chinese medicine**, including **pulse diagnosis** but paying more attention to abdominal diagnosis to determine which points on the meridian require attention. Practitioners may suggest dietary improvements and modifications in lifestyle, and some Western practitioners also incorporate osteopathic and chiropractic techniques into their treatment programmes.

Silva method

A therapy introduced by Mexican therapist José Silva in 1966. It is based on the principle that many people are aware of only the most superficial levels of the mind, and that by using a technique of 'dynamic meditation', which attempts to integrate mind and body using various techniques taken from other well-established therapies, it is possible to contact the deeper levels of the mind, producing relief from stress and tensions.

silymarin /sɪlɪ'mɛərɪn/

A herbal extract from the milk thistle plant, developed in 1968. It is said to have a cleansing and anti-oxidant activity, as well as providing nutrients which help to maintain a healthy liver and protect it from toxins. It has been used to treat hepatitis, cirrhosis of the liver, mushroom poisoning, drug toxicity, and occupational toxic effects. Its actions are not specific to liver cells, although it is excreted by the liver and consequently concentrated there. Silymarin has been shown to stimulate cell protein production and regeneration, to act as a **free radical** scavenger (anti-oxidant), and to inhibit the enzyme lipo-oxygenase, thereby stabilizing the lipid component of the cell membrane.

sitz bath
A treatment requiring two baths with ledges for sitting on, one bath filled with hot water and the other with cold water; from German *sitzen* 'sit'. The treatment consists of sitting in the hot bath for three minutes, with the water covering the hips and abdomen and the feet immersed in cold water. The procedure is then reversed by sitting in the cold water for one minute with the feet in the hot bath; this may be repeated through several cycles. The treatment is said to be good for cystitis, constipation, and haemorrhoids.

smoky quartz
A form of quartz which varies in colour from pale grey to jet black. It is said to dispel negativity and those shadows that prevent one from seeing problems clearly.
See also **crystal therapy**

sociopathology
The study of the sickness of society as a whole and the formulation of possible remedies. The fundamental assumption is that society is based upon erroneous philosophies and organized around corrupt laws which are themselves a major cause of socioeconomic, political, cultural, and scientific problems. These problems are, in their turn, responsible for neurosis, psychosis, and organic illness. Treatment of such illnesses should not just be directed at relieving the symptoms of the individual, but should also include modification of the social factors that produce the illness in the first place.

sodalite /ˈsoʊdəlaɪt/
A deep purple-violet stone which is said to be able to increase spiritual awareness by linking the conscious mind with the

subconscious. It is also claimed to balance the metabolism, lower the blood pressure, and improve the sleep pattern. See also **crystal therapy**

somatids

Ultramicroscopic 'tiny bodies' described by French biologist Gaston Naessens in the 1950s as occurring in the blood of animals, including human beings. They are said to be subcellular, living and reproducing particles which have a distinct life-cycle, divided into 16 stages, that can be interrupted by toxicity or degenerative conditions including cancer, ME, and AIDS. It is allegedly possible, through examination of somatids in the blood, to predict development of these diseases before they actually occur.

somatography

A technique which trains patients in self-awareness so that they can recognize signals from the body, particularly in the form of stresses and tension in muscles. Through these signals patients are able to understand their own thoughts and feelings, as well as receiving early warning of impending problems.

sound therapy

A therapeutic technique based on the use of sound, which has a wide variety of applications in medical and paramedical practice. It includes the use of ultrasound scanners to detect internal pathology, in much the same way as X-rays, and the use of high-intensity sound energy for lithotripsy, which can disrupt kidney stones and gall stones without damage to the surrounding tissues. Low frequency sonic weapons have been investigated for military use, and it has been shown that high levels of environmental noise can cause stress which leads to both mental and physical ill health. Plants are said to grow better when exposed to music, and healing chants and prayers by the repetition of a **mantra** are used in ayurvedic medicine. Each body tissue has its own 'vibration frequency' which may be deranged when diseased, and sound therapy, using tape recordings and electronic devices to generate sounds specific for each tissue, can be applied to the body with the aim of restoring the vibrations to normal. Sound waves may be able to attack diseased cells and strengthen healthy ones, and have been used to accelerate the healing of fractures. Sound therapy is said to be particularly useful for muscle and bone problems such as rheumatoid arthritis, fibrositis, sprains, and myalgia.

See also **ayurveda**

spa

A location where spring water contains minerals or other substances reputed to have healing properties when taken either by bathing in the waters or by drinking them. The name derives from the Belgian resort of Spa, famous for its medicinal springs.

spagyric therapy

A system of diagnosis and treatment developed in Germany and first available in the UK in July 1988, based on the premise that the body fluids (urine, blood, saliva, etc) are unique to each individual, and that analysis of them will reveal information about a person's general pattern of health, as well as about any specific illness present. Samples of blood and/or urine are distilled, separated, heated, and then recombined as a clear liquid. Drops of this preparation are placed on a glass slide, where they crystallize, and the pattern of the crystals is then read. This is said to reveal information about health and disease, including degenerative processes and the presence of external influences such as **geopathic stress**. These methods may give early warning of disease processes before orthodox medicine can detect any changes. The liquid from the recombination process is used to make a **homodot** which is given back to the patient in small doses to stimulate the immune system. The crystalline pattern facilitates the selection of herbs for treatment, and may also be used to monitor response to other forms of treatment.

spiritual healing

A technique of healing, usually transmitted by the 'laying on of hands', and facilitated by specific spiritual practices such as prayer, meditation, or other exercises to concentrate the healing power. The healer (and usually the patient) believe that a supernatural being supplies the healing power, which is channelled through the healer to the patient. Many healers in the West are Christians who attribute their healing powers to Jesus Christ or the Virgin Mary, but most churches do not officially endorse spiritual healing. Although there is a lot of published work about spiritual healing, especially in Russia and USA, there has not yet been a properly controlled study which fulfils orthodox medical criteria. Nevertheless a British Medical Association report in 1956 on 'Divine Healing and Cooperation between Doctors and Clergy' states that 'through spiritual healing recoveries have taken place that cannot be explained by medical science'.

See also **faith healing**

star of Bethlehem

A perennial plant (*Ornithogalum umbellatum*) of the lily family with narrow striped leaves and white flowers from which a **Bach flower remedy** can be prepared. This is said to help those suffering from shock and trauma, both mental and physical, including that of grief and bereavement.

stress

Any factor which has an adverse effect on the body's functioning. The most common stress factors are disease, injury, and worry, and these may affect mind, body, and spirit. Stress reaction commonly results in an increase in muscle tension, which in turn gives rise to headaches, neck and back pain, hypertension, digestive problems, hyperventilation, palpitations, insomnia, anxiety, fear, and depression. Successful people respond to stresses in their lives in a balanced way, and cope with the stresses of everyday life by making the best of each situation, whereas 'victims' fail to adapt to changes and problems. The degree of stress does not correlate directly with the extent of bodily dysfunction, but rather it is the person's own perception of the degree of stress.

subhasrara /səbhəsˈrɑːrə/

The **chakra** which is said to be the bridge with the higher chakras and which connects with the Governor and Conception vessels of the **acupuncture** system of **meridians**. This is the last chakra to be activated by rising energy and through which the human psyche may be transcended.

sublingual drop test
A test designed to identify foods and other substances to which a patient has developed sensitivity. The patient fasts by taking only fluids for five days to detoxify the body, and solutions of foods are then administered sublingually. Symptoms usually develop within minutes, if a sensitivity is present.

succussion
The process by which a homeopathic remedy is prepared. It consists of repeatedly diluting the remedy with a liquid (usually pure alcohol) and shaking vigorously; a fraction of the mixture is then diluted further, and the procedure repeated. The strength of the remedy is expressed as 1 C, 2 C, 3 C etc as each hundredfold dilution and succussion is made. See also **homeopathy; potentization; trituration**

sugalite /ˈʃʊgəlaɪt/
A pink-violet stone which is said to clear the link between the right and left brain and aid development of the third eye or inner vision. It balances the pineal and pituitary glands, and helps children who have learning difficulties, including autism and dyslexia.

suma
An **adaptogen** herb from Brazil where it is known as *para todo* ('for all things'). The active ingredients (pfaffosides) are unique to this plant and are said to support the body's self-regulating processes. The effects of taking this herb are claimed to be similar to those of **ginseng**. See also **pfaffia**

swadhistana /swædhɪsˈtɑːnə/
The second **chakra**, situated at the root of the spinal cord where it is linked with the genital system. It links also with the urinary bladder and kidney meridians, and is said to be

involved with the generative aspect of sexuality — the womb, ovaries, and testicles, and the hormones oestrogen and testosterone.

sweet chestnut

A deciduous tree (*Castanea sativa*) with long catkins from which a **Bach flower remedy** may be prepared. This is said to relieve despair, anguish, and dejection, and to reintroduce hope.

symbiosis

The process by which two different organisms live together and interact together. The term includes *parasitism*, in which one organism exists at the expense of the other, and *commensalism*, in which the plants or animals share their food and do not live at each other's expense.

systematic desensitization

A form of **behaviour therapy** for the treatment of fears and phobias, in which the patient is encouraged to relax and imagine increasingly frightening situations, eventually culminating in full contact and experience of the subject of the phobia.

systematic kinesiology

The science of testing muscle response to pressure in order to detect imbalances and energy blockages. When imbalances are detected, treatment is given by making use of touch, **acupressure**, and diet to restore balance and encourage natural healing. Systematic kinesiology includes all the variations of **kinesiology**, ie *behavioural kinesiology* (BK), *clinical kinesiology* (CK), and *educational kinesiology* (EK).

T

tachyons
Energetic particles which can move through matter and may be converted to human biological energy by their interaction with cell membranes. These particles form the 'gravitational field' and may be the means by which solar flares and **geopathic stress** exert an adverse influence.

tai chi chuan /ˈtaɪ ˈtʃiː ˈtʃuːən/
A composite system of martial art, meditation, and health exercises, the foundation of which is the practice of 'the form', a series of 108 movements each of which has several fighting applications. The 108 movements are practised as a slow flowing sequence which allows the 'players' to harmonize mind, body, and spirit. The origin of tai chi chuan is said to be an encounter between a snake and a crane, observed by a Taoist Monk, Chang San Feng in the 13th century. He devised a series of postures based on the movements of these animals, from which the present forms are developed. The exercises and forms develop, focus, and circulate the **qi** energy through the **meridians**, which also form the basis of **acupuncture** and associated therapies. Tai chi chuan is said to balance the energy flow through the body and mind, and assist in the circulation of body fluids. It is recommended for those suffering tension, anxiety, high blood pressure, and heart problems. An Australian study showed that long term practitioners have greater strength and flexibility scores, with a lower incidence of atheroma, osteoporosis, and spinal deformities than a matched control group. A recent British study has demonstrated benefit in speeding rehabilitation after heart attacks.

taxol
An extract from the bark of the Pacific yew tree (*Taxus brevifolia*), first shown to have anti-cancer activity in a

National Cancer Institute screening programme of the late 1960s. There were initial problems with the trials due to severe toxicity, but nevertheless taxol is said to be the most promising anti-cancer drug developed during the last decade, and it is currently under investigation at the Johns Hopkins University, Baltimore, and other centres. It shows activity particularly against ovarian cancer, and more recently promising results have been obtained in combination with other drugs in the treatment of breast cancer. Unfortunately, it requires the bark from 3 000 trees to make 1 kg of the drug, ie three trees for each patient treated; but attempts are being made to develop a synthetic version.

TCM

See **traditional Chinese medicine**

telepathy

Communication between persons directly from mind to mind, without involving the senses or using any form of ancillary apparatus.

TENS

An abbreviation of *transcutaneous electrical nerve stimulation*, an adaptation of **electroacupuncture** in which surface electrodes are applied to the skin over acupuncture points, and low frequency, square wave, pulsed current is applied. This is a popular technique which for some patients produces effective and prolonged pain relief. It is especially effective for localized and chronic pain, but has also been used for obstetric analgesia and post-operative pain relief. The mechanism of action is similar to that of acupuncture, with release of endorphins into the cerebrospinal fluid and the reticular activating system, and the thalamus may also be involved. It is generally less effective than acupuncture, but has the advantage of being suitable for self-administration. See also **endorphins**

tension

An essential survival mechanism which holds the muscles in readiness for action when danger threatens. Many stresses of moddern living generate tension, but unfortunately for many

people there is no physical release involving muscular activity. The result is a sustained arousal state which may eventually lead to illness or exhaustion.
See also **stress**

teslar 'watch'

A device developed by the Institute of Bioenergetic Medicine in Poole, Dorset, UK, which incorporates an electric coil and microchip, and is claimed to create a protective field around the wearer that neutralizes the extremely low frequency (ELF) electromagnetic radiation emitted by radio, TV, power lines, computers, etc. These ELFs are said to cause nervous system disorders, and to contribute to stress and anxiety.

t-group

An abbreviation of **training group** — a group of 12–20 people assembled for group **psychotherapy** particularly directed at improving their social and working relationships. The group leader may employ specific techniques such as **sensitivity training** or **Rogerian counselling**.

Thai massage

A **massage** technique said to be derived from the methods of Jivaka Kumar Bhaccha, the physician to Buddha, which arrived in Thailand in the 3rd century BC. Various techniques are depicted on 60 stone epigraphs at Phra Chetuphon in Bangkok. The techniques involve using the hands, feet, and elbows to work on the body's 'healing energy lines', which are similar to the **acupuncture meridians**. This mobilizes the patient's own natural healing energy. The method also incorporates stretching, bending, and pulling movements.

thalassotherapy

The use of the healing powers of sea water and/or seaweed. These may be used as a compress, as a poultice containing vitamins, minerals, and trace elements, or in baths, where the buoyancy of the sea water gives support to allow the exercise of stiff and painful joints.
See also **hydrotherapy**

therapeutic touch

A form of healing in which the therapist first clears the mind by visualization or meditation to allow free flow of psychic energy, and then lightly places the hands over any areas where sickness or imbalance are detected, thereby allowing healing energy to flow and restore balance. The technique is popular in the USA.

thrush

See **candida**

tibb

[Arabic, 'nature'] A system of health care developed in the Middle East and which combines elements of traditional Chinese and Indian medicine with Greek and Arabic medicine. In this system health is viewed as a state of wholeness and balance. Diagnosis is a holistic assessment of the individual, attempting to localize the source of any imbalance. Treatment includes **massage, manipulation, psychotherapy**, and **herbal medicine**.

tiger's eye

A yellowish-brown form of **quartz**, used as a gem because of its brilliant lustre, and said to concentrate and focus physical energy. It brings thoughts and imaginings down to earth, helps to develop insight, encourages good luck, and purifies the body after over-indulgence.
See also **crystal therapy**

TIM

An abbreviation for **traditional Indian medicine**; see **ayurveda**.

tincture

[Latin *tingere* 'to stain'] An alcoholic herbal extract prepared by adding 40% spirit to ground or chopped dried herbs. Spirits such as vodka or gin may be used as the source of alcohol. The resulting mixture is left for two weeks with regular mixing before decanting, which results in a long-lasting and concentrated extract of the herb. This should be taken in small doses.

tisane /tɪˈzɑːn/

[Latin *ptisana* 'barley, barley water'] A preparation drunk for medicinal purposes. It is often sold in the form of tea bags, and the term can be applied to any weak herbal tea used in this way.

tofu

[Chinese *dou* 'bean' + *fu* 'curdled'] A form of bean curd made from soya bean, widely available in health food shops, and a frequent component of oriental cuisine and macrobiotic diets. It is virtually tasteless, and so is usually served steamed, boiled, or fried with seasoning, sauces, and vegetables.

See also **macrobiotics**

tolerance

The process by which the body becomes accommodated to the presence of addictive substances, and then requires increasing amounts of the substance to maintain the same effect. This may be the result of a change in the way in which the substance is metabolized in the body.

tongue diagnosis

A fundamental examination technique of **traditional Chinese medicine** in which the appearance of the tongue is analysed according to its colour, shape, coating, and the presence of any surface markings such as cracks or ulcers. The assessment includes noting whether the tongue is moist or dry, swollen or shrunken, and still or quivering. Particular areas of the tongue are said to be related to specific internal organs, and surface features on the tongue may reflect disease processes affecting the related organ.

tonoscope

An instrument developed by Dr Hans Jenny which produces a three-dimensional visual image of sound. The sound of 'O', for example, is depicted as a perfect sphere by the instrument.

See also **sound therapy**

topaz
[Hindi, 'fire'] A transparent and lustrous gemstone form of
aluminium silicate, which is either white, yellow, pale blue, or
pale green in colour. It is said to bring light into life, protect
against danger, relieve stress, and encourage sleep.
See also **crystal therapy**

touch for health
A modified form of **kinesiology**, developed by American
chiropractor John Thie and colleagues in the 1960s, which
combines the use of muscle testing to assess imbalance with
the principles of **traditional Chinese medicine**. Treatment is
based on the use of **massage, acupuncture**, and light touch by
brushing along the length of affected acupuncture **meridians**
to release blockages and restore energy flow.
See also **chiropractic**

tourmaline
[Sinhalese *toramalli* 'carnelian, mixed colours'] A silicate
gemstone usually pink and green in colour, claimed to
facilitate the movement of consciousness between different
levels and to eliminate misunderstandings and intolerance. It
is a balancing stone which has a calming effect, encourages
communication and cooperation, and is reputed to help heal
a broken heart.

traditional Chinese medicine (TCM)
A system of medicine developed in China with origins dating
from c.5000 BC, and based on the meticulous observation of
natural phenomena related to patterns of disharmony
affecting the human mind, body, and spirit. Some of the
fundamental principles relate to Taoist philosophy. Health is
seen as the harmonious balance of **yin** and **yang** energy, and of
the mind, body, and spirit. Disease may be due to internal or
external 'perverse energies', named according to the climatic
variations that they resemble, such as wind, heat, and damp.
Disease in an organ leads to abnormal energy flow in its
associated channels, and treatment is designed to correct
stagnation and blockage of this energy flow, thus restoring
normal function. The major bodily functions are attributed to
the five **zang** organs or 'solid organs' (heart, lung, kidney, liver

and spleen), each of which is linked to a hollow **fu** organ. The emotions are also governed by specific organs. Diagnosis is based on a detailed history and a clinical examination which emphasizes the *eight principles* and *four methods*, including **pulse** and **tongue diagnosis**. A TCM diagnosis can be used to formulate treatment using various techniques such as **acupuncture, moxibustion, aromatherapy, shiatsu** and **herbal medicine.**
See also **perverse energy**

traditional Indian medicine
See **ayurveda**

Trager psychophysical integration
A technique of non-invasive bodywork developed in the present century by American physician Elton Trager to help the victims of poliomyelitis and other neuro-muscular disorders.

transactional analysis
A technique of **psychotherapy** developed by Canadian psychiatrist Eric Berne (1910–1970), who wrote the best-selling book *Games People Play* in 1964. A 'transaction' is a unit of communication between players of the 'game'. A 'script' is the life plan that we live out from decisions which we make in childhood. Clients learn about their games and scripts and see how they are employing 'childhood strategies' in their adult life, and use this understanding to intepret their own life patterns and their ways of relating to other people. This may cause them to change their behaviour.

transcutaneous electrical nerve stimulation
See **TENS**

transmitter crystal
A crystal with a three-sided pyramidal face which can transmit or direct healing energy, or communicate feelings of love, to family or friends who are far away.

trichology

[Greek *tricho* 'hair, comb'] The study of the structure, function, and diseases of the human scalp and hair. The condition of the hair may reflect general health, including stress, tension, lifestyle, and variations in other body systems. Hair analysis has been used to assess the body's mineral status, including the presence of poisoning by heavy metals.

trigger points

Specific points, which may correspond to acupuncture points or to sites of local tenderness, used to treat more widespread musculo-skeletal pain, sometimes in areas remote from the trigger point itself. These points may be stimulated by acupuncture, injection, **massage**, or heat.

triple heater

One of the **yang** organs described in **traditional Chinese medicine**. It has no actual counterpart in Western anatomy, but rather describes a collection of functions concerned with the circulation of **qi**. The three 'heaters' are also said to correspond to three zones of the body: the *upper* heater, above the diaphragm; the *middle* heater, between the diaphragm and the umbilicus; and the *lower heater*, everything below the umbilicus.

trituration

The preparation of a homeopathic remedy by grinding the substance in a bowl to produce an intimate mixture with a solid carrier substance (usually lactose). One part of this mixture is then added to another nine parts of carrier, and the procedure repeated to the required potency in the same way as a liquid dilution.

See also **homeopathy; potentization; succussion**

tsubu

The surface points along **meridians** which correspond to **acupuncture** points, and which are pressed or massaged during **shiatsu** treatment to stimulate the flow of **qi**.

tui na
A Chinese system of remedial **massage**, dating from the Han period, which is designed to sedate by 'thrusting and rolling' hand movements.
See also **an mo**

Turkish bath
A form of steam bath, the heat from which is too moist to allow the evaporation of sweat. This produces very heavy perspiration which is believed to remove body impurities, but which may be dangerous for patients with circulatory problems.

turnip
An annual or biennial vegetable (*Brassica rapa*) with an edible tap root, which has been used as a poultice, either raw or mashed up with bread and milk. It is also used in East Anglia to produce a cough syrup by heating with brown sugar.

turquoise
A bright blue-green form of aluminium phosphate, regarded as a semi-precious stone which symbolizes the sky and the spirit. It is said to give courage, strength, and power, and to be good for the lungs and respiration.
See also **crystal therapy**

U

ultrasonics

A technique using sound with a frequency of greater than 20 000 Hz, which is undetectable by the human ear. It can be produced by vibrating a quartz crystal at very high frequency in an electric field, and pulses may be used to treat muscle strain and sports injuries, to relieve pain, and also in a scanning device to produce an image of the internal organs and tissues which can be constructed by computer from the echoes that result from the reflection of the sound waves back through different tissues. This has been especially applied to monitor intrauterine growth and development, and has become a useful alternative to X-ray, particularly of the abdomen and pelvis.

umeboshi plums

Pickled sour plums, usually added to cereal or vegetable dishes, rather than being eaten alone. They are said to be good for settling the stomach.

unani tibbia /jʊˈnɑːnɪ ˈtɪbɪə/

A traditional form of medicine which originated in Greece but was then taken to India by the invading Turks in the 7th century AD. It still survives in Delhi at the Hamdard Institute. The principles of diagnosis are similar to those of **traditional Chinese medicine** with an emphasis on feeling the pulse. Treatment relies mainly upon herbal remedies, and advice about diet and life style.

V

vega

An electrical device which can record a patient's electrical resistance when a probe is placed on an **acupuncture** point. Test substances (eg allergens or remedies) can also be incorporated into the circuit, and the apparatus is said to be able to detect disturbance of the internal organs, **geopathic stress**, vitamin and mineral deficiency, the presence of poisonous or therapeutic substances, and to help in the selection of homeopathic remedies. The results seem to depend as much upon the operator as upon the subject, and the use of the apparatus could perhaps best be regarded as a form of **dowsing**.

See also **homeopathy**

vegan

A person who is a strict vegetarian, eating no meat or any other animal product. This gives a diet that is low in fat and high in fibre, and which, although basically healthy, is deficient in minerals such as calcium, iron, zinc, and vitamins, especially B_{12}. It is usually necessary to provide these missing factors in the form of dietary supplements.

vegetotherapy

A form of treatment by **manipulation** based on the theories of Austrian psychoanalyst Wilhelm Reich (1891–1957), who believed that the presence of emotional problems resulted in unnatural breathing patterns and muscular tensions, especially in the abdomen. The tension, and consequently the emotional problem, is said to be relieved by this form of manipulation.

vervain

A perennial plant (*Verbena officinalis*) with spikes of lilac flowers from which a **Bach flower remedy** can be prepared. This is said to promote relaxation and relieve the tension and frustration which result from overenthusiasm.

vibrasound

An electronic system for integrating music, sound, and light into a 'sensory resonance' which is said to allow one to see, hear, and feel the music. This is claimed to promote relaxation, relieve stress, improve health, well-being, creativity, memory, and learning.
See also **sensory resonance**.

vine

A deciduous woody climbing plant with numerous tiny green flowers from which a **Bach flower remedy** can be prepared. This is said to enable those who are arrogant and domineering to be more understanding and tolerant of those weaker than themselves.

violet

The colour of change and transformation, associated with the crown **chakra**. Violet people are often creative and spiritually conscious, but tend to be unworldly and live in fantasies of their own.
See also **colour therapy**

vishuddi /vɪʃʊdi/

The fifth **chakra**, situated in the neck and linked with the throat, where it connects with the vocal cords and vocal expression and also with the ears and the function of hearing. Some say that it corresponds to the Western thyroid gland, and that it produces the 'nectar of immortality'.

visualization

A process which involves making a deliberate attempt with the conscious mind to create mental images. These images may be closely linked to emotions, and can induce sensations and actual physical changes. Creative visualization of beneficial and health-promoting images can have positive effects which help to promote natural healing processes.

vitamins

Organic substances required in minute amounts by the body, which are esssential for health and generally control the way in which the body uses other nutrients. Some are water soluble (eg vitamin B complex and vitamin C); others are fat or lipid soluble (vitamins A, D, E and K). Vitamin D is produced by the action of sunlight on the skin, and vitamin K is synthesized by gut bacteria, but all the other vitamins are required as essential micronutrients in the diet, and deficiency leads to illness. If the diet is deficient, for example in strict vegetarians, alcoholics, the elderly, or in pregnancy, vitamin suppplements are necessary to maintain health.

voice therapy

A series of vocal and breathing exercises sometimes used together with **massage** and **psychotherapy**, designed to establish a connection between the voice control centre and the emotions. This enables those who cannot control the tone, pitch, or rhythm of their voice to express their emotions appropriately. Inappropriate vocal expression sometimes follows physical disability or may be due to acquired behaviour patterns, such as in conditions of anxiety or depression.

voice work

A broad description of the various ways, such as singing, chanting, breathing techniques, and bodywork, which enable people to work upon their vocal sounds and to increase their range of expression by allowing them to use their voices more fully. It is useful for those who lack confidence or who find it difficult to express themselves.

Voll apparatus

A device devised by German acupuncturist Reinhard Voll which can measure the charge at an **acupuncture** point. This is said to reflect health or disease at the point or in its related meridian and internal organs. A practitioner using this apparatus can diagnose internal disease and apply treatment by adjusting the altered charge back to normal.

See also **meridians**

W

walnut

A deciduous tree (*Juglans regia*) which produces catkins from which a **Bach flower remedy** can be prepared. This is said to help people through periods of transition in life, such as marriage, divorce, puberty, and the menopause, and also to avoid diversions from one's chosen path.

water birth

A technique of child birth pioneered in the 1960s by Dr Igor Tjarkousky and then taken up and developed by French obstetrician Michel Odent (1930–   ) at Pithiviers Hospital in France. The technique involves conducting the last stage of labour using a water birth pool containing enough water at near body temperature (35–37°C) to reach the armpits when seated (ie 38–40 cm in depth). The warm water encourages relaxation and eases labour pains and movements. This is said to reduce the duration of labour and the incidence of foetal distress, and to reduce the need for episiotomy and pain-killing drugs.

water violet

A perennial plant of the family *Violaceae* with five-petalled flowers from which a **Bach flower remedy** may be prepared. This is said to help those who are quiet, reserved, isolated, and lonely. The remedy enables them to be friendly to others without compromising their privacy.

whole body therapy

A form of cancer treatment developed by Dr Joseph Issels at the Ringbert Klinik in Germany. Nutritional supplements and immunotherapy are used to build up the body's own defences, so that they can be an effective complement to orthodox treatment including surgery and radiotherapy.

See also **immune system; nutritional medicine**

wholism
An anglicized spelling of **holism**.

wild oat
A type of cereal of the family *Gramineae*, from which a **Bach flower remedy** can be prepared. This is said to help those who wish to see their way ahead more clearly, particularly when at a crossroads in life.

wild rose
A genus of shrubs and scrambling perennials of the family *Rosaceae*, with five-petalled flowers which may be white, yellow, red, or purple, from which a **Bach flower remedy** may be prepared. This is said to revive the emotions and vitality of those who are drifting aimlessly through life and becoming disinterested and apathetic.

willow
A deciduous tree of the family *Salicaceae*, which forms catkins from which a **Bach flower remedy** can be prepared. This is said to help people who have a negative attitude to life and have become bitter and self-pitying. The remedy is said to encourage a positive and optimistic outlook.

withdrawal
Symptoms which affect drug addicts when an addictive substance is not available to them. Addicts become dependent on the presence of an addictive substance which enters the body's biochemical pathways and may alter the body chemistry. When this substance is withdrawn, the body responds by producing *withdrawal symptoms* which include nausea, vomiting, stomach cramps, anxiety, panic attacks, palpitations, headaches, insomnia, hallucinations, shaking, sweating, and even convulsions. Curing drug dependency usually involves giving diminishing doses of the addictive substance, and imitating its biochemical effects to minimize the withdrawal symptoms by using similar, but less addictive, substances. The addict must have a genuine desire to stop taking the drug, and **counselling** and other kinds of support

are required to maintain this motivation. Many self-help organizations (eg Alcoholics Anonymous) are available for this purpose.

See also **addiction**

wrapping

An empirical form of treatment which is said to be good for skin disorders, bronchitis, and chronic backache. A sheet is soaked in cold water, wrung out, and applied by wrapping around the body. A dry sheet and a warm blanket are then wrapped over the top of the wet sheet, and the patient remains in the wrap until the wet sheet dries out before finally towelling dry.

wu chin hi /'wu: ʧin 'hi:/

A system of physical exercise otherwise known as 'the Game of the Five Animals', invented by the surgeon Ha To who lived in the Han dynasty (approximately 200 BC). *Niao-hi*, the 'bird game', improves breathing; *yuan hi*, the 'monkey game', teaches climbing, and the other animals represented are tiger, stag, and bear.

wu cycle

A way of depicting the interrelationship between the **five elements** and a mechanism for dealing with imbalance between them which acts in the reverse way from the **ko cycle** or 'controlling sequence'. The wu cycle is otherwise known as the 'humiliating' or 'counteracting' sequence in which, when expressed in terms of the elements, wood counteracts metal; metal counteracts fire; fire counteracts water; water counteracts earth; and earth counteracts wood.

See also **sheng cycle**

X, Y

xenobiotics
Foreign chemical compounds which may have toxic effects when absorbed into the body.

xenoglossia
See **reincarnation**

yang
One of the two complementary but opposing forces which divide 'the void' and form the foundation of Taoist philosophy; the other being **yin**. In **traditional Chinese medicine** good health exists when yin and yang balance each other, and ill health is the result of an absolute or relative deficiency of either yin or yang. Yang is the positive male force, which is aggressive, stimulating, light, hot, and dry. Yang also refers to the exterior or surface of the body and the back. The yang meridians take their origin from the yang organs, which are the stomach, **triple heater**, gall bladder, bladder, colon, and small intestine. Yang people tend to be active, alert, energetic, and precise, but suffer from tension, irritability, and inability to relax. Yang foods have warmth, energy, and strength (eg meats, eggs, cheese, brown rice, bean stews).

yellow

A warm colour which expresses joy and happiness and is associated with the intellectual side of the mind and the solar plexus **chakra**. Yellow persons tend to be good organizers but are often moody.

See also **colour therapy**

yin

The complementary and opposing principle to **yang**. It represents the flexible, fluid, cooler, side of nature which includes cold, dark, negative, and female. Yin represents the interior and the front of the body. The yin meridians emanate from the yin organs, which are the liver, heart, spleen, lung, and kidney. Yin people tend to be calm, relaxed, peaceful, and creative, but are also prone to lethargy and depression, and have difficulty in concentrating. Yin foods have a calming, cooling, and relaxing effect (eg tropical fruits and juices, raw vegetable salads, steamed fruits, steamed vegetables).

yoga

[Sanskrit, 'unity (with life and the divine)'] A way of life which provides a personal system of health care and spiritual development and emphasizes the harmony of mind, body, and spirit. There are various schools and styles of practice with a variety of physical and contemplative techniques, including:

mantra yoga — which employs chanting and vibrations;
karma yoga — which encourages self-development by service to others through work;
bhakti yoga — which employs religious love and devotion;
laya kriya yoga — which uses sexual relationships to achieve bodily and spiritual fulfilment;
hatha yoga — which is concerned with health through mastering the body, using a series of precise postures (*asanas*) each one comprising body movement, mental control, and breath control paying particular attention to the diaphragm.

The practice of yoga has been shown to benefit a wide variety of problems, including hypertension, arthritis, dysmenorrhoea, and stress-related problems. Special classes for handicapped people have reported wide-ranging benefits, including increased flexibility, relaxation, and improved concentration.

yoghurt

A popular dairy food product which results from the action of bacteria (*Lactobacillus bulgaricus* and *Streptococcus acido-philus*) on milk to produce lactic acid, which partly curdles the milk resulting in a gelatinous consistency. Live yoghurt is sold with the **acidophilus** bacteria still alive, which is supposed to reinforce the natural flora of the gut. In heat-treated, UHT, pasteurized, or sterilized yoghurt, all the bacteria have been killed. Low fat yoghurt contains less than 2% fat, whole milk yoghurt contains 3.5% fat, and Greek yoghurt contains 10% fat.

Z

zang

A collective term used in **traditional Chinese medicine** for the solid organs which are governed by the **yin**. These comprise the kidney, lung, liver, heart, and spleen.

See also **fu**

Zen

A form of Buddhism which originated in India and then spread to China, where it was influenced by, and incorporated some principles of, Taoism. Zen was introduced to Japan by monks returning from China in the 12th century. It is characterized by an emphasis upon personal experience of enlightenment by direct insight into one's self through meditation, mindfulness, and simple living, without the need for complicated rituals.

zero balancing

A system of **bodywork** developed by American physician Fritz Smith, who claims to have developed methods of palpating stress-induced changes in the structure and energy of the musculo-skeletal system. The body can then be encouraged, using techniques related to **acupressure** and **osteopathy**, to rearrange itself into a state of harmony or 'balance'.

zone therapy

A technique, devised in 1913 by American ENT surgeon William Fitzgerald, which divides the body into ten surface zones, of equal width, each relating to specific parts of the body. Applying pressure with the hands, or with instruments, to the appropriate zone is said to relieve pain in the related parts.

See also **reflexology**

APPENDIX
INDEX OF ABBREVIATIONS

A

ACET	Aids Care, Education and Training
AHPP	Association of Humanistic Psychology Practitioners
AIPTI	Association of Independent Professional Therapists International
AIRMT	Associate of the International Register of Manipulative Therapists
AMA	Anthroposophical Medical Association
AMP	Association of Massage Practitioners
AMTA	American Massage Therapy Association
ANLP	Association for Neuro-linguistic Programming
ATA	Associate of Tisserand Aromatherapists

B

BAc	Bachelor of Acupuncture
BAAR	British Acupuncture Association and Register
BAAT	British Association of Art Therapists
BAC	British Association of Counsellors
BAHA	British Alliance of Healing Associations
BALCT	British Association of Lymph and Colon Therapists
BATHH	British Association of Therapeutic Hypnosis
BCA	British Chiropractic Association
BCHE	British Council of Hypnotherapy Examiners
BCNO	British College of Naturopathy and Osteopathy
BH	Bachelor of Humanities (University of London)
BHFTA	British Health Food Trade Association
BHMA	British Holistic Medical Association
BIEMS	Bio-Electromagnetic Society
BMAS	British Medical Acupuncture Society
BNOA	British Naturopathic and Osteopathic Association
BPS	British Psychological Society
BPSS	British Society of Psychotherapists
BRICCAP	British Congress of Complementary and Alternative Practitioners
BRS	British Rebirth Society
BSD	British Society of Dowsers
BSO	British School of Osteopathy
BWOY	British Wheel of Yoga

C

CAc	Certificate of Acupuncture (China)
CAHF	Campaign Against Health Fraud
CCAC	Certificate in Chinese Acupuncture
CCAM	Council for Complementary and Alternative Medicine
Cert HS	Certificate in Herbal Studies
CHO	Confederation of Healing Organizations
CHP	Certificate in Hypnotherapy and Psychotherapy
CHip	Council of Hypnotherapists
CMH	Council of Master Hypnotists
CNAA	Council for National Academic Awards
CO	College of Osteopaths
COET	College of Osteopaths Educational Trust
COMA	Committee on the Medical Aspects of Food Policy
CQSW	Certificate of Qualification in Social Work
CRRO	Confederation of Radionic and Radiesthetic Organizations

D

DAc	Diploma in Acupuncture
DC	Diploma in Chiropractic
DHM	Diploma in Holistic Medicine
D Hom	Diploma in Homeopathy
CHP	Diploma in Hypnotherapy and Psychotherapy
Dip BWY	British Wheel of Yoga Diploma
Dip C	Diploma in Counselling
Dip Hyp	Diploma of Hypnotherapy
Dip PC	Diploma in Psychic Counselling
Dip Phyt	Diploma in Phytotherapy (Herbal Medicine)
Dip THP	Diploma in Therapeutic Hypnosis and Psychotherapy
DO	Diploma in Osteopathy
D PM	Diploma in Psychological Medicine
Dr Ac	Doctor of Acupuncture
DSH	Diploma from the School of Homeopathy
D Th D	Diploma in Dietary Therapy
DTM	Diploma in Therapeutic Massage

E

ECIM	European Council for Integrated Medicine
ECPM	European Council for Plurality in Medicine
EFNMU	European Federation of Natural Medicine Users
EHPM	European Health Product Manufacturers Federation
ENT	Ear, Nose and Throat
EOTA	Essential Oils Trade Association
ESO	European School of Osteopathy

F

FBAcA	Fellow of the British Acupuncture Association
FBRA	Fellow of the British Reflexology Association
FFHom	Fellow of the Faculty of Homeopathy
FIHP	Fellow of the Institute of Hypnosis and Para-psychology
FRH	Fellow of the Register of Herbalists
FNTOS	Fellow of the Natural Therapeutic Osteopathic Society

G

GCRN	General Council and Register of Naturopaths
GCRO	General Council and Register of Osteopaths

H

HFMA	Health Food Manufacturers Association

I

ICAK	International College of Applied Kinesiology
ICM	Institute for Complementary Medicine
IFA	International Federation of Aromatherapists
IFPNT	International Federation of Practitioners of Natural Therapies
ISPA	International Society of Professional Aromatherapists
ITEC	International Therapy Examination Council

J

JACM	Journal of Alternative and Complementary Medicine

L

LLCH	London College of Classical Homeopathy
LCH	Licentiate of the College of Homeopathy
Lic Ac	Licentiate in Acupuncture
LLSA	Licentiate of the London School of Aromatherapy
LNCP	Licentiate of the National Council of Psycho-therapists and Hypnotherapy Register

M

MAA	Member of the Auriculotherapy Association
MAC	Master of Acupuncture
MACH	Member of the Association of Classical Hypnotherapists
MAHPP	Member of the Association of Humanistic Psychology Practitioners
MAPT	Member of the Association of Professional Therapists

MAR	Member of the Association of Reflexologists
MARC	Medicines Advisory Research Committee
MBAcA	Member of the British Acupuncture Association
MBEOA	Member of the British European Osteopathic Association
MBNOA	Member of the British Naturopathic and Osteopathic Association
MBRA	Member of the British Reflexology Association
MBRI	Member of the British Register of Iridologists
MBSA	Member of the British School of Acupuncture
MBSH	Member of the British Society of Hypnotherapists
MBSR	Member of the British School of Reflexology
MC	McTimoney Chiropractor
MCA	Medicines Control Agency
MCH	Member of the College of Homeopathy
MCO	Member of the College of Osteopaths
MCOA	Member of the Cranial Osteopaths Association
MCROA	Member of the Cranial Osteopathic Association
MCSP	Member of Chartered Society of Physiotherapists
MFG	Member of the Feldenkrais Guild
MFHom	Member of the Faculty of Homeopathy
MFPhys	Member of the Faculty of Physiatrists
MGO	Member of the Guild of Osteopathy
MH	Master Herbalist
MHPA	Member of the Health Practitioners Association
MIACT	Member of the International Association of Colour Therapists
MIAH	Member of the Institute of Analytical Hypnotherapists
MIFA	Member of International Federation of Aromatherapists
MIIR	Member of International Institute of Reflexology
M Inst AT	Member of the Institute of Allergy Therapists
MIPTI	Member of the Independent Professional Therapists International
MIRMT	Member of the Independent Register of Manipulative Therapists
MIROM	Member of the International Register of Oriental Medicine
MISPH	Member of the International Society for Professional Hypnosis
MISPT	Member of the International Society of Polarity Therapists
MNAHP	Member of the International Association of Hypnotists and Psychotherapists
MNCP	Member of the National Council of Psychotherapists and Hypnotherapy

M Rad A	Member of the Radionics Association
MNIMH	Member of the National Institute of Medical Herbalists
MPNLP	Neurolinguist Programming Master Practitioner
MRCHM	Member of the Register of Chinese Herbal Medicine
MRCN	Member of the Register of Clinical Nutritionists
MRH	Member of the Register of Herbalists
MRN	Member of the Register of Naturopaths
MRO	Member of the Register of Osteopaths
MRSH	Member of the Royal Society of Health
MRSS	Member of the Register of the Shiatsu Society
MRTA	Member of the Relaxation Therapy Association
MRTCM	Member of the Register of Traditional Chinese Medicine
MSAAc	Member of the Society of Auricular Acupuncturists
MSAPP	Member of the Society of Advanced Psychotherapy Practitioners
MSBM	Member of the Society of Biophysical Medicine
MSHP	Member of the Society of Holistic Practitioners
MSS	Member of the Shiatsu Society
MSTAT	Member of the Society of Teachers of the Alexander Technique
MTAcS	Member of the Traditional Acupuncture Society
MWFH	Member of the World Federation of Hypnotherapists

N

NAHS	National Association of Health Stores
NCC	National Consultative Council (of Natural Therapies)
NCVQ	National Council for Vocational Qualifications
ND	Diploma in Naturopathy
NFSH	Natural Federation of Spiritual Healers
NIM	Northern Institute of Massage
NMG	Natural Medicines Group
NMS	Natural Medicines Society
NRHP	National Register of Hypnotherapists and Psychotherapists
NVQ	National Vocational Qualification

P

PGCE	Post-Graduate Certificate of Education

R

RCCM	Research Council for Complementary Medicine
RGN	Registered General Nurse
RIR	Registered Iridologist
RMANM	Registered Member of the Association of Natural Medicine
RMAPC	Registered Member of the Association of Psychic Counsellors
RMN	Registered Mental Nurse
RPT	Registered Polarity Therapist
RSHom	Registered with the Society of Homeopaths
RTCM	Register of Traditional Chinese Medicine

S

SAPP	Society of Advanced Psychotherapy Practitioners
SHIP	Self Help in Pain
SRCh	State Registered Chiropodist
SRN	State Registered Nurse
SRP	State Registered Physiotherapist
STAT	Society of the Teachers of the Alexander Technique

T

TDHA	Tisserand Diploma in Holistic Aromatherapy

W

WFH	World Federation of Healing
WOPACM	Working Party on Alternative and Complementary Medicine